TAPS identical twins and COVID

A story of surviving

Nichola Luther

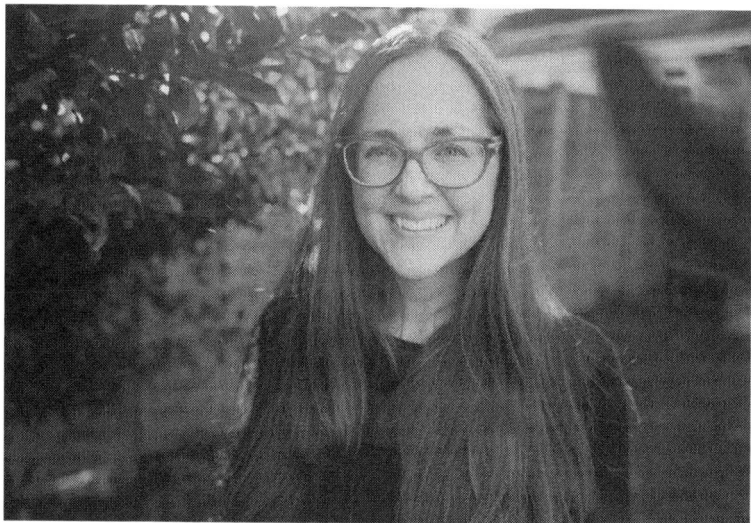

Nichola lives on the Isle of Wight with her three gorgeous boys and husband Pete. This is her first book.

For more information and pictures see
www.tapstwins.co.uk

This book is dedicated to all the amazing health professionals in fetal medicine and Neonatology, involved in saving our babies' lives. St George's Hospital, Tooting. Princess Anne hospital, Southampton. St Mary's hospital, Isle of Wight.

Especially to Professor Asma Khalil and Dr Raji Parasuraman.

We will be forever grateful.

Acknowledgements

Thank you

Tom Fallick for the incredibly beautiful cover.

Professor Asma Khalil for writing a wonderful foreword, fact checking and believing in me.

Gemma Calloway for spending your precious time reading and copy writing for me. I couldn't have done it without you.

Nosy Marketing for having faith in me; particularly my dear friend, Lorraine Lawton-Berry, and Henry George for your unending support and kindness.

Reuben Mowle for the beautiful photos.

Matt Smithers for coming on board and taking on the challenge with me.

Twins Trust for allowing me the use of the graphics, writing articles and all the amazing support and help.

Philippa Harper at St George's for all your support and advice.

Stephanie Ernst, at Taps Support, for always being there and understanding everything.

My family, as always, for their constant love and support, I love you all dearly.

Contents

Foreword

This is a wonderful book; it is beautifully written and very moving—I thoroughly enjoyed reading it. Nichola provides such a wonderful, personal insight into the trials and tribulations that parents, babies, and their families have to go through in these challenging circumstances.

Twin Anaemia Polycythaemia Sequence (TAPS) is a rare condition affecting identical twins. Nichola's account of her twins' TAPS journey provides parents and families with invaluable information about this condition, and its implications. But this book is more than that—it also beautifully describes the emotional journey that parents and families of babies in the neonatal unit have to navigate, regardless of the reason they need that care. I believe that this book will be valuable for, and valued by, any parents going through the 'neonatal unit emotional roller-coaster.'

Professor Asma Khalil—Professor of Obstetrics and Maternal Fetal Medicine at St George's Hospital, University of London.

Introduction

Why would you want to read a book about taps... they just produce water, don't they? Yes, but this book is actually about Twin Anaemia Polycythemia Sequence (TAPS) and the fight for our identical twin boys to survive. Add in the World Covid Pandemic, and you can begin to imagine how a horrific situation became so much harder.

This book isn't all sad though: I'm going to tell you our journey; highlight TAPS; talk about giving birth during a pandemic, and mention all things neonatal (and how COVID really made the turd unpolishable!) My husband didn't even get to meet the boys until they were 4-and-a-half weeks old, and I didn't hold my babies until then either. However, our two glorious twin boys survived and completed our family, so I think it's important to share this story.

Let's start there.

Our family consists of me, Niki Luther, my husband Pete, our wonderful 3-year-old Sebby (potty training, too!) and our twins, Asher and Leo. As I write, the twins are now 10 months old (7-and-a-half months corrected) and gorgeous!

We live on an island called the Isle of Wight, which is situated three miles from Portsmouth. It's beautiful here, but not the easiest place to get off quickly when you need a specialist hospital during a world pandemic.

All I will say is: a helicopter makes an appearance later in the book!

"It's twins!"

Finding out we were expecting twins was certainly a crazy experience. I'd had a fairly normal start to the pregnancy, but with horrendous morning sickness (whoever called it morning sickness is quite frankly mad! Everyone suffers differently, some hideously.) I had twenty-four-hours a day of feeling like I wanted to puke my guts up, from five weeks pregnant until twenty weeks pregnant. Even the word "ginger" made me dry heave (yes, it is meant to be good for sickness... blurrrr). People tell you: *'Just think of the bundle in your arms at the end,'* and, *'the worse the sickness the healthier the baby'.* However, when you're in the middle of what feels like a permanent sickness bug, you don't feel quite so positive or cheery!

I was quickly getting much bigger than I did with Sebby. Second pregnancy can do this, so I didn't think much of it.

I also have a condition called hypothyroidism, which is fairly common and treated for life with a drug called Thyroxine. This meant that—along with my geriatric status (*41 in November...yes, you are considered 'old' when expecting at this age. It does mean you get extra care, although I'm not talking Tena ladies and falsies...*)—I was seen at six weeks pregnant by the consultant endocrinologist. My levels were closely monitored throughout. During the first twelve weeks of pregnancy, the baby/babies don't make any thyroxine, so they take the Mummy's. It's very important there is enough, otherwise (amongst other complications) it can cause miscarriage.

12 Weeks Pregnant

I was due a 12 week scan in a week's time. However, following a spot of bleeding, I was seen straight away on the 3rd December, 2019 (St Mary's Hospital, Isle of Wight). Pete and I were very nervous and scared, hoping the baby would be ok. I can remember the sonographer's face: I instantly knew something was different.

I asked if all was ok and she answered: "More than ok!"

The sonographer turned the screen to face us, "There are two babies and they both have healthy, beating hearts!"

I instantly burst into tears and hysterical laughing. Pete was white and shocked. The sonographer then had a good look and informed us I was about 12 weeks along, carrying identical twins. The sonographer knew this because- as far as she could see- the twins shared a placenta, but had separate sacs. They call this monochorionic (Latin for one placenta) diamniotic (meaning two-sacs) twins.

I was then booked an appointment for the following week for a longer scan and an appointment to see the specialist, who would tell us exactly what this entailed. We were told it was a high-risk pregnancy and I would be needing a lot more care.

On an interesting note, identical twins aren't genetic meaning they don't run in the family. They occur when the fertilised embryo splits and creates two genetically identical small humans—it truly is a miracle! Out of every 1000 pregnancies, there are around twelve twin pregnancies. Then out of all twins born, around one third are identical (so out of a million births, that's around 4000 identical twins).

We went away in shock to work out our feelings, and to tell our parents and Sebby.

13 Weeks Pregnant

The following week we had another scan and saw the consultant. She confirmed that I was indeed carrying identical twins and I was now roughly 13 weeks, 6 days. We were in there for about an hour as the consultant provided the nitty-gritty.

My pregnancy was high risk. I would need to be scanned every two weeks (from 16 weeks) to check the growth of the babies—and more, if there was any concern. This was mainly to do with something called Twin to Twin Transfusion Syndrome (or TTTS for short,) which can occur when the babies share a placenta.

In TTTS, there is a donor baby and a recipient baby: the latter takes all the goodness (oxygen, nutrients etc.) Basically, recipient baby 'eats all the pies' and doesn't allow the other baby to grow properly, which—without treatment—can result in losing one or both twins. It's serious if you get it, and treatment is needed to improve their chances. It can be diagnosed as early as the first trimester, twelve weeks. They monitor you regularly to check for changes in size and other factors that could suggest TTTS is happening.

The consultant also explained that, whatever happened, I would be giving birth at 36 weeks. However, she stressed that most twins come early, so it really is a week-by-week plan. If our babies came before 34 weeks, I would be delivering at the Princess Anne hospital in Southampton. If there were any worries at all, I would be going straight over to Southampton. The babies would very likely go straight to Special Care Baby Unit (SCBU) at St Mary's on the island, or neonatal at Princess Anne— depending on their birth date.

We had a due date of June 15th and a birth date of May 18th. The consultant did stress that hopefully everything would be fine, and that I would be constantly looked after. Everyone was lovely, kind and excited about having twins born. I was already anaemic and B12 deficient, so the doctors started me on both iron and B12, as well as pregnancy vitamins. They said they would be checking my thyroxine levels regularly, as well as needing a gestational diabetes check at 26 weeks. This is due to age and a multiple baby pregnancy. My lovely midwife joked that I may as well pitch a tent outside, as I'd be here a lot (little did we know about the journey that lay ahead...)

I was given various pamphlets on this, that, and the other. Pete and I went home in a little bit of a blur. Not only did we need all of this to sink in, but we were going to be the parents of three under three!

- *Sidebar: it took us a long time to conceive Sebastian. We weren't sure we were able to at one point, but with the twins it was instant. We later joked it took two hundred tries for Sebby, and one for the twins! They were certainly very much a miracle in lots of ways. Sebby was also a very "normal pregnancy" (apart from some of my health issues, which were controlled—another topic for another time). Sebby came along at 39 weeks plus 5 days. He did need forceps and I needed an episiotomy, but he came out crying after twenty-eight hours (very exhausting but normal for first baby) of labour. We were then in hospital for a week (not quite so normal), as I'd had Group Strep B, a benign bacterium that one in five women carry in their bodies. (It lays dormant and generally causes no harm to us, but can occasionally be problematic for the baby.) He needed to be monitored for twenty-four hours. His infection levels went up and he needed antibiotics and was then put on a special light machine, as he became extremely jaundiced. It was a scary week and I remember shuffling around the hospital with my clean sanitary towel in one hand, and a jug in the other, going between maternity, SCBU and the toilet. Once you have a baby, all cares and worries of any dignity go completely out of the window. I remember it being very frightening and exhausting, but the staff were amazing and we got through and came home stronger for it, with a very healthy Sebastian! I'm going to go into neonatal/ SCBU later. It definitely helped having had this small encounter with the island SCBU: I felt I had a little more understanding of what might happen, and I was a little less scared.*

First sign of a problem

16 Weeks Pregnant

We had our 16 week scan on December 31st, where we excitedly found out we were having boys! We would know for definite at the next scan in two weeks' time. Everything looked ok.

18 Weeks Pregnant

We returned on the 14th January for our two-week check. This involved measuring each baby's head, tummy size and length of leg (putting this into very clever technology gives the sonographer an idea of size). They also checked each baby's bladder (it is another sign of TTTS if no bladder is present, if it's empty, not visible or a lot smaller). They checked the size of the fluid in the two sacs to check both babies had roughly equal amounts. All seemed ok with both babies, apart from their sizes, which were showing a 22% difference. If it's above 20%, this is when they start to look closer. After speaking with the consultant in Southampton, they thought they'd monitor in the first instance.

20 Weeks Pregnant

Two weeks later, the size difference was 29%. Two days later, on January 30th, we were seen by the Fetal Medicine team at the Princess Anne Hospital in Southampton. This appointment was fairly positive.

Again, they saw no sign of TTTS and they thought the size difference was ok for now. They were happy to see me four-weekly, with the Island hospital seeing me in-between.

We were sat down in a side room after the scan and given a clear explanation by the consultant, a specialist doctor, and a fetal midwife about what would happen if the size difference continued. I would need to be seen more in Southampton and it was very unlikely that the pregnancy would go beyond 34 weeks. Getting to 32 weeks is the aim for these type of twins, as they are more likely to be early. I was told that I may even have to be admitted early to be monitored if problems persisted or arose. Lastly, they explained that—given all the complications—it would probably be a planned Caesarean, but again they wanted to get the pregnancy as far as possible. The longer the babies stayed in, the more chance they would have to survive.

The babies would most likely be delivered in Southampton. There were no real 'definites,' except that, at some point, these babies would decide to enter the world... or have that decision taken away from them.

We went home with many thoughts. We were glad all seemed ok, but we also realised that the road ahead could become 'bumpier.' We were slightly baffled by all the 'what ifs.'

My biggest worry at this point was my gorgeous two-year-old, Sebby. *How would he cope with his Mummy being on the other side of the water? How would I see him? How would Pete still work?* I couldn't stand the thought of us being parted. Up until this point, Sebby had been my world. I'm lucky enough to be a full-time mummy, so Sebby and I had spent all of our time together, and he was very much a mummy's boy. I was terrified about how we would cope being separated! I didn't want to leave my baby. *Would we get accommodation at the hospital?*

So many thoughts.

I'm a born worrier, so it was hard for me not to get carried away with the 'what ifs,' but I tried to focus on 'the now' and growing my babies. I was feeling a lot better in myself. The sickness went just after Christmas, and apart from getting tired, I was able to enjoy my Sebby, and being pregnant again.

Then it all changed.

TAPS

24 Weeks Pregnant

I had reached 24 weeks! In my mind, that was a real goal. It meant that my pregnancy was more viable, and my babies had a better chance of survival if born early. We had our four-weekly check up on the 25th February; this time with a different consultant, who was just as thorough as the consultant before. She checked the sizes: all seemed ok. Hearts: all ok. Bladders: present, and ok. Water in sack: even, and plenty of it.

As the babies were now 24 weeks, they checked something called their Middle Cerebral Artery levels (MCA). This is basically measured from an artery in the brain and it shows how effectively the blood is pumping around the babies' bodies. I could tell something wasn't right instantly because it was like watching a wave on the screen and I could see that they were very different in both babies. The consultant was also checking it again and again, and talking to the fetal midwife about what she was finding. We knew something could be wrong, but she wanted to explain properly once the scan was over and we were seated in the room next door. I remember her coming in... I think the midwife was there too, possibly even another doctor. She explained our babies had very different MCA levels: it looked as though Asher wasn't getting enough blood, and Leo was getting too much. This would also mean Asher's blood would be thin and he would become anaemic, which would then lead to heart failure. Conversely, Leo's blood would be very thick (Polycythemia), which would mean it pumped around his body more slowly. This could lead to other problems, like blood not reaching his extremities to grow.

These were the symptoms of a condition called Twin Anaemia and Polycythemia Sequence (TAPS).

It occurs due to the babies sharing a placenta. One baby becomes the donor and one becomes the recipient of the red blood cells. The consultant explained that, at present, our babies weren't showing signs of distress, and it was possible that it wasn't going to get any worse. She felt no action was needed just yet, but that she would need to see us in a week to check again. In the meantime, she would speak with St George's Hospital in London to get their fetal surgeon's opinion. She went on to say that spontaneous TAPS was very rare: they had never had a case at Southampton. There was currently no cure for it, but there were certain procedures they could do at St. George's that could help reverse it.

The syndrome has only been known for about 15 years, so there is still not enough research on it. There are not enough cases to really know the outcome, why it happens, and how to prevent it (or cure it). At this stage, she was very hopeful that it wasn't TAPS and the levels wouldn't get worse. There are two forms of TAPS: Spontaneous TAPS, and post-laser surgery TAPS, which is a complication of TTTS laser surgery. I've since found out that the statistics show 3-5% of monochorionic twins can get TAPS: that's 3-5 babies out of 100 monochorionic twins who may get it, which shows how incredibly rare it is. However, due to it being such a new disease, data and research is still not available to give completely accurate figures. The numbers could be a lot more.

With this in mind, she said we must try not to worry (yep, that's not going to happen!) and keep growing those babies. She did go a little more into viability, explaining that, because they were twins (and my babies specifically were very small), the stats of survival are lower than with a single birth. Generally, if the babies were further along and a problem like this arose, then they would just deliver and treat the babies outside of the womb. Once outside, syndromes like TTTS and TAPS stop deteriorating. We were given all the paperwork to show us 'weeks' and 'outcomes.' It became more apparent how important it was to keep the bubbas in to help them grow. I think the consultant was hoping it wouldn't progress past stage one or two, or it wouldn't be TAPS, and that the babies would stay fairly stable. Hopefully, we'd just need weekly monitoring and then— once viable (or if showing distress)—the babies would be delivered.

TAPS has five stages. Intervention is needed from stage three, and by stage five it's too late for one or both babies.

As you can imagine, there were a lot of tears, but again we had to focus on the fact that it was probably ok. My two-year-old was waiting in the car with my Dad, so after a quick explanation to Dad, we did what any parent must do with a young child... carry on! In fact, we went to IKEA. It's funny the ordinary things you do in extraordinary circumstances.

I found the following week hard. I was very teary and emotional a lot of the time. I just didn't know what was going to happen. I'd been told not to *Google* TAPS as it wouldn't help, especially where it was so rare: fifteen-years this year! (*There isn't a lot online about it, and what's there is very scary.*) Unfortunately, I didn't listen. I'm sorry, but you tell me my babies might have some horrific disease and it's very hard not to get *Safari* up! True to word, there wasn't a great amount of information out there and certainly no positive stories that I could find. A lot of it was research-based facts for people in the know, so was very hard to make heads or tails of. There were no bullet points or anything I could grab hold of, just a lot of scariness.

One of the reasons for writing this book is because I never want another parent to go through this. I want someone to find that story of hope I had: someone to know they are not alone. I want other parents to be given the information in a way that a parent can understand. I never want someone else to have to go through what we did. Fairly recently, when doing some research for this book, I found some sites with helpful information: I will mention these later in the 'facts and terms' section. It shows how much can change in a year.

25 Weeks Pregnant

The following Monday, 2nd March, we were back at the Princess Anne in Fetal Medicine. It was just Pete and I,

26

leaving Sebby with my parents back on the IOW. We were very nervous, and unfortunately the MCA levels had gotten a lot worse. It was definitely spontaneous TAPS. We were again sat in the side room. I was inconsolable and Pete couldn't believe this was happening. The staff were so kind to us: the consultant just kept saying sorry.

We were told that the consultant had spoken with St. George's (London) and they wanted us to go there today or tomorrow, calling us first. The fetal team may decide to do laser surgery straight away or continue monitoring. It would depend on what stage they thought the TAPS was at. It looked as though it could be developing quickly, and once the babies showed signs of distress, we could lose one or both of them. Again, we heard all the grisly statistics; the rarity of the condition; the small size of the babies; the lack of research and cure.

They have to keep it real. The team want you to be positive, but they need you to know it's a very uncertain fight ahead with the potential for a sad outcome.

The team made sure that we were in the best hands. We were being sent to the best fetal surgeons in the country: if anyone could save the babies, it would be them.

It's funny to reflect now: at our very first consultant's meeting at 13 weeks, St. George's was mentioned for extreme circumstances… and here we were, having reached those. We were the 3%. *Why us?*

St. George's

That afternoon, we got the phone call asking if we could arrive first thing tomorrow: Tuesday 3rd March. If we booked a 7am ferry, then we could be up in London by 10.30am. St. George's is in Tooting, London, so it's a pretty straight forward journey up the A3 from Portsmouth. They told us to get to them as soon as we could and they'd be waiting. My mind was hazy; the tears were constant. My mum and dad were with us so they helped pack. We'd been told to bring an overnight bag in case they needed me to stay in.

Sebby must have been very confused: I made sure to cuddle him lots. He was going to have to stay with my parents for the night, or even two. It was the first time he'd ever been away for the night, and that in itself was a big step and an emotional one. My brave boy went off and was amazing. Pete and I tried to rest and get our minds ready for the morning. At this point, COVID was very much in the news, but hadn't affected our little island yet. Travelling hadn't yet changed, so we used the ferry as normal. (This was to change very quickly over the next week.)

We were at the ferry terminal by 6.30am the next morning. The ferry journey from Fishbourne to Portsmouth was only around forty minutes, and the drive to the hospital only took us an hour and forty minutes; the traffic was kind to us. We tried to make the journey as comfortable as possible. At 25 weeks, my bump was nearly the size of full-term with Sebby. The twin babies had decided to push up into my ribs, and any mummy who has experienced this knows it feels a bit like your ribs are breaking (it only gets more uncomfortable if you can't change position a lot!) Being in a car was not the best, but plenty of snacks and a pregnancy pillow kept me going—with toilet breaks, of course!

We actually arrived at 9.30am, but it took us half-an-hour to park. We tentatively took our first steps into the hospital to find Fetal Medicine. Once there, we weren't sat for long when the midwife came to get us. We were first ushered into a side room and met our wonderful surgeon, Professor Asma Khalil. She wanted to know everything about our case so far, and what we'd been told. Until she scanned us, she didn't want to make any assumptions as to if it was TAPS yet.

We were also asked if we minded being filmed. Channel Four were filming a documentary to highlight rare cases that the fetal surgeons dealt with daily. *Did we mind being filmed?* At this point, we were kind of living a nightmare, so it was surreal and unexpected to be asked this. However, it gave us something different to focus on. The film crew were lovely and stressed that, at any point, they could stop. Pete and I decided we were happy for them to go ahead, providing we could stop if we needed to, and say no at any time. We knew how rare and serious this disease was: if we could help other parents not have to go through what we were, then yes please.

We went in for the scan. The consultant very quickly confirmed the awful truth that yes, it was spontaneous TAPS. Additionally, the MCA levels were rapidly getting worse. Leo had what they called a 'starry liver,' and Asher was showing signs of cardiac distress. This was advanced TAPS and, if something wasn't done, then one or both babies would die. Back into a side room we went, and the consultant talked us through everything. She explained again what TAPS was, but in greater detail. Again, she was so sorry that we had to go through this: there was no cure, but we had three options (the babies were just too small to deliver).

Number one: Laser Surgery. Surgeons would go into the womb to try to sever the arteries in the placenta that were joining the babies. This would try to stop Asher from giving Leo all of the red blood cells.

Number two: a blood transfusion in the tummy to help Asher.

Number three: do nothing and hope that—as it's so rare—it may correct itself. This was not an option for us.

We asked for the surgeon's opinion, and she felt that (although there was no definite) laser surgery was the best option for a chance of survival. If the laser surgery wasn't successful, we still had the option of a blood transfusion. We were then left to talk it through.

It is hard to describe how you feel when the worst happens. It's like you go into a vacuum, a bubble, and you can't believe what's happening. You're having to

make life and death decisions about your unborn babies.
In that instant, there's no definitive answer. At the same
time, something clicks in. I think it's our human will to
survive; to beat the odds; to know that curling up in a
ball won't help. You have to keep going; you have to
keep strong for the babies, and push forward. Despite my
constant tears, that's what we did.

For me, information is power. I like to know everything. I
ask questions: it makes me feel better. I wanted exact
explanations of what might happen and what were the
odds. I was like this right from the start of the
pregnancy.

Pete and I put our trust in these amazing surgeons. It
was the babies' best chance. As Asher was so poorly, the
surgery had to happen very quickly so we were checked
in straight away. Surgery was booked for the next
morning. Our surgeon explained that I would be awake
throughout and would be given a local anaesthetic in the
spine, which basically makes you numb from the boob
down. It's very much like an epidural used for labour or a
Caesarean section. She also warned us that there would
be a lot of people in the room. Two reasons: one, it was
a teaching hospital; two, it was such a rare case that it
was important for other members of the fetal team to
watch. There would also be the film crew. Once the
operation was over, the most important thing was that
the babies stayed put! The first twenty-four hours after
surgery, it was crucial that I didn't go into labour.

Talking of the film crew, they were with us the whole
time; asking how we felt, wanting to know the process.

It's crazy being filmed when you're going through something so horrendous. I was letting people see us so raw. The film crew saw my pain but, at the same time, I think it helped. It gave me and Pete something else to focus on. We were able to think about letting people know how we felt, so that—in turn—it might help them. I think it was very much like therapy for us... being able to talk, and being so supported. Everyone was just so kind and so amazing.

I was checked into a ward and told to rest as much as possible. There were blood tests done and stats taken (blood pressure, temperature). We then had to try and find Pete some accommodation. There was no free accommodation and Pete wasn't allowed to stay overnight. At this point, the hotel attached to the hospital was still open. With help from our midwife, we were able to secure a room. It wasn't cheap, but what else could we do?

The rest of the afternoon I mainly rested. We phoned home to explain what was happening—*that* was very hard. We had to explain to Sebby that we would be away for at least two more nights, but we tried to keep it as upbeat as possible. Luckily, he was having a fabulous time with his grandparents, so I think it was more painful for us! I'd never been parted from him. As soon as my mum was alone on the phone, I broke again: *why us? Why was this happening?* It must've been so hard for family 'watching on.' All they could do was support us, and wait.

From this point, another way I dealt with the pain and grief was to shut down and keep myself cocooned, apart from Pete, Sebby, Mum, Dad and Pete's parents. I physically couldn't talk to anyone else, as I knew I wouldn't be able to control the hysterical tears: reliving the pain (every time I had to tell someone what had happened) was too hard, emotionally. It was very important to keep as calm as possible for the babies. Too much upset would not be good for any of us. Instead, I wrote group messages to keep my amazing family and friends up-to-date, as they were all so concerned and supportive. It was lovely to know how much they cared. To this day, I don't think some of them realise how much their daily messages of support meant to me in the subsequent weeks! It kept me going, especially when I was alone (this will be explained later).

Pete had to leave around 8pm, which was horrible! I didn't sleep at all that night. Apart from pregnancy being uncomfortable, I was just so nervous about the next day; I really needed Pete. I held it together all night until around 5am. I was exhausted and scared. Luckily, Pete was back in by 6am.

Operation

They prepped and had me ready to go for an 8.30 am start. I remember having to walk from the ward down to the theatre in my gown, being followed by Pete, the film crew, and our midwife. She kept telling me she wasn't going to leave my side—and she was true to her word! It was very surreal! Some of the lifts weren't working, and the others were very busy, so they asked me to use the stairs if I felt able, which I did. Several people went past us… I don't know what they thought of a heavily pregnant woman with a film crew coming down the stairs!

When we reached the theatre, it was like watching the 'parting of the sea' as we moved towards the door. Everyone knew we were the 'TAPS patients.' *The rare case.* Everyone had sympathetic eyes, with kindness emitting from them. It was all very strange and surreal considering we were fighting for our babies' lives; it was a very weird bubble to be in. I was so scared, but I knew I just had to be brave and get on with it.

True to word, the theatre was packed: Pete and I think there were around thirty people! There were the fetal surgeons, anaesthetists, nurses, doctors, student doctors, consultants, and the people who looked after the equipment (to make sure it all ran perfectly) and, of course, the film crew! There was certainly no room for shyness! That said, I kept my focus on the task ahead, so I didn't really notice at the time.

The theatre was very nice. There were even painted flowers on the ceiling for something to focus on whilst laying there! I was looked after by two anaesthetists and a nurse, who gave me the spinal anaesthetic, and observed me throughout. They were very funny and lovely. A spinal anaesthetic goes into your back: you have to hold very still whilst they numb the area to insert the needle, and then they use a very cold spray to check that the anaesthetic is working. Everything below has to go numb before they can begin. Any heavily pregnant lady can relate to feeling very uncomfortable, but once that spinal tap works, you feel nothing. It was the first time in months I had actually felt comfortable: no pain!

We had both of the top fetal surgeons in with us, Professor Basky Thilaganathan and Professor Asma Khalil, who would be performing the operation, as well as another consultant. Throughout my time with the Fetal team, and then into Neonatal, I've come to admire the sense of humour these people have! It's amazing how they manage to make you feel relaxed and laugh, despite the horrific situation. *They are the kindest people, who genuinely want to make you feel at ease. You feel safe with them. Equally, baby surgeons are very special, intelligent, funny, kind people who have dedicated their lives to saving tiny babies. They are truly amazing (and very well dressed, might I add!)*

The operation lasted about an hour, and Pete held my hand the whole time. We could have watched on the screen, but I just focussed on the ceiling! I was keeping calm and getting through. The anaesthetists spoke to us the whole time, as did my midwife. Once the laser was turned on, everybody had to wear protective goggles, so we had a room full of people basically wearing sunglasses! Again, very surreal. Apparently, on the screen, you could see a red baby and a white baby, showing how poorly the babies were. The baby surgeons worked hard: they had to find the arteries in the placenta (connecting the babies) and then block or cauterise them using a laser. To do this, they had to sedate the babies and then exchange fluid in one of the sacs, so they could see the placenta with a camera. The procedure had to be very precise. (Fetal surgeons really are amazing: the skills they need to do this are so finely honed and tuned. It's miraculous in itself!)

The operation was over. I was wheeled to recovery. I would have another scan, later that afternoon, to see how the twins had responded. We could already tell from the surgeons' reaction that the operation had gone well. They put a Glyceryl Trinitrate (GTN) patch on my tummy to try to stop any contractions over the next twenty-four hours, and told me the most important thing was to rest and keep the babies in.

Later that afternoon, we went for the scan. As you can imagine, we were both very nervous. The amazing thing was that both babies were responding well with their vital signs. No change yet with the MCA levels... but no change was good—they were no worse. The consultant said the operation had gone better than they had hoped. I would have another scan in the morning and then hopefully we would be able to go home, and be back again the following week. She already explained that it was likely that the MCA levels wouldn't change a great deal for a couple of weeks, so we mustn't worry too much. The important thing was to see that they weren't deteriorating, and hopefully we would start to see a slow improvement. In the meantime, we must keep those babies inside, so they could have a really good chance to recover and heal. Both babies were still far too small to survive being born.

The next morning was the same. The scans showed the babies' vital signs were better, but the MCA levels were still the same. Again, this looked positive. We had a scan booked for exactly a week later, then drove home. The drive was quite uncomfortable, but I just focused on getting home to see Sebastian.

The next week was hard. Physically, I was swollen, aching and exhausted from the laser surgery and travelling. Emotionally, I was deeply, deeply saddened and scared by the situation—despite trying to remain hopeful and positive. I just wanted my babies to live. Apart from my immediate family, I still couldn't speak to anyone else. I couldn't handle the pain, and knew that— for the babies' sake—I needed to keep as calm as possible. Their chances of survival would be better with healing time, so they needed to stay put, and I needed to rest.

My parents and Pete's parents were amazing! They took over the running of our house and supported Sebby and I, whilst Pete was at work. Although I was there with constant cuddles and love for Sebby, our parents did the practical things. I really needed my mum, and I was lucky enough to have her around.

The next three weeks

26 Weeks Pregnant

I haven't mentioned much about Covid yet. Despite the Covid pandemic getting worse around us, it was the least of our worries at the time to be honest. The previous week, an islander had tested positive for COVID after travelling on a Wightlink ferry—the same day we'd used the ferry to travel to St George's! The island now had its first positive case and our small, generally safe island was under as much threat as the mainland UK from the awful virus.

By the following Thursday, we were off early to London again. Physically, I felt much better, but emotionally, I still felt all over the place. During the ferry journey, we were allowed to stay in the car as we were deemed very vulnerable. At this point, masks weren't mandatory: plenty of handwashing and gel was the advice. We also decided not to go into any service stations because of the risk, so we hilariously decided to wee into an ice cream carton in the car when we could find a discreet place to stop. We even used Sebby's potty at one point! For a heavily pregnant woman, this was interesting to say the least.

Once we reached the hospital, the film crew met us at the car. They'd become invested in us, in the same way that a close friend would be, and genuinely wanted to keep in contact and check we were okay. They'd been through it all with us. Filming commenced as we reached Fetal Medicine and we were taken straight through. Again, the kindness and safety of the fetal team enveloped Pete and I in a bubble of hope. We were nervous, but I'd felt the babies moving so I had hope that they were still alive.

During the scan, my gorgeous bubbas were wriggling around happily: their vital signs were good; their hearts perfect. We also found out that there was the smallest of changes to the MCA levels (nothing dramatic, but enough to think it could be going in the right direction!) Due to all other vitals being good, the consultant felt no other interventions were needed at this stage. Again, the message was to 'keep the babies inside,' rest as much as I could, and they would scan me again the following Thursday (19th March).

Another week went by. Covid was getting worse and I was feeling even more vulnerable. I was starting to worry with Pete at work. Pete runs a charity called 'Revive Newport.' Within this, he has a community café (The Living Room) and a youth café (NYC). This worry was taken out of our hands from Tuesday 17th March onwards. Pete had to close the cafe and work from home. The start of restaurants and cafes shutting down due to Covid had begun.

We had to sit down with our parents at this stage and have a frank discussion about how we would handle the situation. How would we look after our gorgeous Sebastian, if Pete and I were making weekly (if not more) hospital visits? Plus, there was the very real possibility of going into labour at any point! Due to Covid, Sebby couldn't be with us for any of this. We needed to know that he would be safe, and this meant protecting us and the babies too. The only option was for us, my parents, and Pete's parents to begin shielding completely. We already knew that Sebby would stay with my parents when I went into labour, but we needed to know both sets of parents would be there to look after him and help me out up until then, and after. This meant that none of us could see anyone outside of our bubble: this included Pete's sister, my brother and any friends. We were so grateful that they all agreed to make this sacrifice for us. Little did we know that, only a few weeks later, everyone else in the UK would be in the same situation...

27 Weeks pregnant

We headed up to St George's again on the 19th March (we stayed in the car and used another ice cream carton!) Everything became harder the bigger I was! Again, we were met by the film crew. This time, everyone was masked up and the fetal waiting room was pretty empty as appointments were now spaced out. Only absolute necessities were being seen for other scans. Again, the babies' vital signs were good, as were their hearts. They were growing well.

The MCA levels were again slightly changing for the better, so all was looking positive. We had reached 27 weeks, 3 days. It was a few more days to get to the 'golden 28 weeks,' where the babies would have better chances of survival if born. The twins were still very small, so every day counted. We booked to come back the following Thursday, and at that appointment we would also have an MRI to see how the babies' brains were. We'd be at the hospital all day.

It is—as yet—unclear what neurological damage spontaneous TAPS can cause. It is known that, especially for the donor twin and some recipients, they do suffer to some effect. We had to pray that our boys were both okay and that, despite their illness, their brains had still developed. One of the other documented side effects of TAPS is deafness, but that couldn't be tested until the boys were born. At that moment in time, we just hoped for two babies born alive. The rest we could deal with. We had another long journey home, and more rest to 'keep those babies in.'

Another blow

28 Weeks Pregnant

The UK government stipulated the country's first lockdown on Monday 23rd March, 2020. This meant everything, apart from essential shops and medical needs, had to close. Even schools.

We all had to stay home. Covid-19 was on the rampage.

On Tuesday 24th March, I had my gestational diabetes appointment at the local hospital, St. Marys. I found it very emotional: it was the first time I'd returned to the department and seen my midwife since the operation, so I found it very hard to talk about it all. There were a lot of tears. The maternity staff were so supportive and pleased to see me, which helped a lot.

When you go for a gestational diabetes check, you can't eat anything from when you wake until it's finished. You go in first thing and get given a special drink, then have to wait two hours before they test your blood sugars. Due to being over forty and carrying multiples, I was eligible for the test; it was only meant to be a precaution. It was lucky that I did attend, however, because I was later informed that I did, in fact, have gestational diabetes. I was asked along to the diabetes clinic the next morning to talk about the treatment. It was another blow to my already difficult pregnancy.

Due to Covid restrictions, I was the only person being seen at the clinic; it was shut to anything other than emergencies. The treatment for gestational diabetes is mainly diet-led, alongside regular blood testing. I had to have a low carbohydrate and sugar diet. At the start, I had to take my bloods first thing in the morning, then just before (and an hour after) every meal, plus at bed time.

This totalled around eight times a day, then after five days reduced to six times, before and after meals. I'd have to do extra testing if I was feeling poorly at all during the day. This was to constantly monitor any changes, and then address them if needed.

If controlling gestational diabetes with diet isn't successful, then you are given metformin tablets to help; if they don't work then it's insulin injections. I was given a kit which explained exactly what I needed to do. On top of everything I'd been through so far, some of my favourite treats were now a big 'no.' There would be no real 'comfort eating' for me, plus it was just another thing I had to monitor. It was a little upsetting.

On a positive note, I am coeliac, so I'm used to dietary issues. As a child, I wasn't allowed sugar, dairy, yeast, amongst many other allergies and intolerances for many years (another story) but in some ways this helped, as I knew what to do and how to look after myself. With a bit of reading up on carbohydrates, too, I made a good food plan to get myself through.

By the end of the day, I felt better about things with my plans in place. Unfortunately, that wasn't quite the end of my day...

28 weeks plus 3 days Pregnant

I went to bed as normal. We had to be up in time for the 7am ferry to travel back to St. George's for our third scan since the laser surgery. Sebby had gone to my parents for the night.

I noticed a little more fluid in my sanitary pad (I'd been having to wear sanitary towels anyway and, to be honest, I just thought I'd wet myself a little—probably wishful thinking on my part!) I really didn't want anything else to go wrong, so I went to sleep.

At 5 am, I woke up wet through and it was obvious that my waters had broken. I didn't have any contractions, but I knew I was uncomfortable and we needed to get somewhere quickly! Our babies were still only 28 weeks, 3 days. They would need to be born on the mainland if possible as, at this stage, they would definitely need Neonatal Intensive Care Unit (NICU). Pete and I were a bit muddled. We didn't know who to call as we were being treated by three different hospitals: we were meant to be going to London in a couple of hours, but knew our birthing hospital would be Southampton. *Where should we go*?

After frantic phone calls, we were sent straight to our local hospital, St Mary's, who would then get us transferred. The priority was to get us in 'medical hands' as soon as possible, and St Mary's was a fifteen minute drive away. If these babies came, their only chance of survival would be in professional care. The babies could arrive quickly where they were still so small.

Once there, the wonderful midwives at St Mary's looked after me brilliantly. I still wasn't having contractions, so they needed to get me transferred to the mainland as soon as possible for the care we needed. However, this involved finding somewhere that would take us. We needed two cots in neonatal, and a free bed in antenatal. Ideally, we needed to be in Southampton, but if they couldn't take me, then anywhere with a fetal medicine department was good. Initially, Portsmouth's Queen Alexander Hospital had two cots, but no beds in antenatal (so they could take the babies, not me). Luckily, minutes later, Southampton got back to us and they had space.

We needed to get there quickly. The ferry wasn't an option, as it would take too long, so a helicopter was called. It was actually the Coastguard helicopter that appeared for us! It was all very surreal. Pete joked that he didn't know whether to be extremely worried or excited, because he was getting to ride in an awesome helicopter! It did make us smile, despite being in a horrendous situation. I was a ticking time bomb. *(I later found out that the hospital staff nickname antenatal patients 'the ticking time bombs'—they just don't know who will explode first, and when!)*

The coastguard team were amazing. The hospital initially strapped me to a gurney, but when the coastguard leader arrived, he very quickly decided I should be unstrapped. He thought it would be best that I could move and lie or sit however I wanted. Comfort was more important. We were wheeled through the hospital to the helipad and myself, Pete, midwife, coastguard and all our luggage was loaded onto the helicopter. It was a twenty minute flight, and if the situation had been different, it would have been an incredible experience. Truthfully, it was already dawning on me that I had two babies who needed to stay put, and I was helicoptering away from my two-year-old, with no knowledge of when I might get to see him next. I just tried to focus on getting to the Princess Anne Hospital; all other thoughts were a bit too overwhelming in that moment.

Southampton March 26th 2020

Once we arrived at Southampton General Hospital's helipad, the ambulance took me over the road to the Princess Anne and straight to their Labour ward. I was instantly strapped up to a Cardiotocogram (CTG) machine to monitor the babies' heart rates, at the same time as measuring for any contractions. The staff measured my heart rate and checked my stats regularly, too.

By this time, it was 11am. I still wasn't registering any contractions, but they wanted to keep me in the Labour suite for twenty-four hours before transferring me to a bed in the antenatal ward. They also wanted me to be scanned as soon as possible in Fetal Medicine; to check the babies MCA levels; to see how their TAPS was, and to check their growth.

It was a very scary situation with the babies. I just kept thinking and saying: 'they are not ready yet, they need to stay in; they are too small. I can't lose them...I've come so far.' I wanted my babies.

Plus, I now realised that I wasn't going home and, due to COVID, Sebastian wasn't going to be allowed to visit me, so I had no idea when I would see him again! My precious baby boy—'my everything' up until now—was now across the water from me. The thought of not seeing him for another day (let alone weeks or months) was just horrifying. Imagine thinking that you may not see your two-year-old for three months! How much they change in that time… everything I would miss. I wouldn't hold him; I couldn't cuddle him or be there for him. How could he understand that I hadn't just abandoned him? It broke me. It still does now, thinking about it. I couldn't control the crying: I wanted my Sebby with me.

This was the first major blow from COVID. We always knew it would be difficult because of the stretch of water separating us, but at least I'd have been able to see Sebastian and my parents as often as possible. Now, I couldn't see any of them, and it was a waiting game as to how much longer Pete would be able to stay with me. He was allowed in the Labour suite, as we had a private en-suite room, but antenatal was an ever-changing situation. We just had to hold on to the fact we were together now. As usual, the midwives were so kind and couldn't do enough for us: you could see it broke their hearts to see the situation unfolding.

At this time masks were being put on, then taken off. The COVID situation was changing hourly, with different stipulations on the hospital, staff and patients.

That afternoon, we were seen at Fetal Medicine. We were going to find out if the boys' TAPS was improving. This is when our first miracle happened. Both boys were looking happy and all vital signs were good! As for the MCA levels, they were nearly back to normal. We couldn't believe it! It meant that, if the babies were born right now, they had a greater chance of surviving from TAPS, at least.

However, they were both still very small—not even two pounds each—so every day counted towards getting them bigger. The fetal consultant really didn't think the babies were coming today, but they erred on the side of caution by keeping me in the labour suite overnight, then moving me up to antenatal the following morning. I would definitely need to stay in until the babies were born because my waters had broken but, providing I kept infection-free and the babies' vitals remained stable, then we could potentially go until 32 weeks (at least). The longer they stayed in, the better.

I was booked in for a fetal scan the following Thursday, and then an MRI on the Friday. The MRI was the one we were meant to have at St. George's to see if the TAPS had left any neurological brain damage. I would need at least two CTGs a day to keep an eye on the babies (CTGs measure a baby's heart rate, which indicates if the babies are still happy and detect any contractions), and otherwise bed rest.

Back in the labour suite, it dawned on me yet again that I could potentially be without Sebby for up to twelve weeks, and I was heartbroken. I struggled to hold it together every time I *FaceTimed* him as the pain was too much. My baby boy… I wanted him with me! Thank goodness for modern technology (although getting a two-year-old to speak on *FaceTime* was easier said than done). On top of this, there was the ever-nearing threat that Pete would soon not be allowed in the hospital. As it stood, he still was, so we held onto that. He was allowed to stay overnight in the labour suite, but once on the antenatal ward, he would have to go home in the evening.

Due to Covid, all the housing available to parents and families of long-term patients were being closed down, so we had no free accommodation available. We searched through 'Airbnb' to find some affordable, private space that Pete could stay for now. It needed to be safe, as we needed to shield as much as possible. It was all very expensive, and for some people, it just wouldn't have been manageable. Our saving grace was the fact that we had just taken out more money from our mortgage for the house and twins, so we had to use that. The alternative would have been for Pete to head back to the island, but that would mean he wouldn't make the birth, and we just didn't know when or how that was going to happen. I was still the ticking time bomb.

We knew that Sebby was being looked after, and that he was happy with his amazing grandparents. He just thought he was on holiday, so we decided Pete needed to stay near or with me. We found somewhere within twenty minutes walking distance of the hospital, and booked Pete in for the following few nights until we knew what was happening. Luckily, I didn't go into labour over the next night, so I was transferred to a private room in antenatal on Friday 27th.

On the ward

Once admitted to the ward, I was put on antibiotics to fight any infection that could occur from my waters having broken. This was standard procedure. The trouble was, I'm allergic to quite a few antibiotics and other medicines, so the doctors had to find an appropriate prescription that would be strong enough to fight any infection, yet I wouldn't react to. This meant phone calls back to the island for lists, and then me needing to remember various names. It became a bit of a joke with the midwives! Every time I had any medication, I had to recite back everything I was allergic to (it was hard to remember). I got quite good at it in the end. *I can't remember any of it now though (I like to blame baby brain!)* I also had to take anti-sickness tablets to help keep the antibiotic down.

A word of caution to all new mums-to-be (especially of multiples)—pack your hospital bag early!

Pete and I had managed to scramble together a few bits when my waters broke, but in all the panic, I forgot to pack pants! On top of this, I just didn't have enough clothes to see me through for potentially three months, and no way of washing, due to COVID. We had to get my mum and dad to go to our home and pack for both myself and Pete. Pete's mum then came across on the ferry and dropped our belongings to the hospital. *Our parents are amazing!*

Things with Covid were still changing within the hospital. Now all staff had to wear masks, and we were all needing to constantly wash and gel our hands after every movement outside of our room or when meals were sent etc. I had my regular CTG, and otherwise, I rested.

Where my waters had broken, I was constantly leaking large amounts of fluid (new fluid is made every day). I was finding my tummy would increase in size daily, and then I would have another massive leak, as there was nothing keeping the water in. My tummy would deflate: it was a very strange feeling. The one upside was the intense pain in my ribs was easier as the water leaked out. I was constantly having to change pads to keep dry and infection-free.

My CTGs were quite hard work. It was a long process to get both babies' heart beats for at least twenty minutes, consistently. Leo decided to skip out of ear shot a lot and so broke the reading. Sometimes, I would be attached for maybe two hours, just to get the right reading. It wasn't painful. I had a probe to track any contractions, and then two others to track each baby's heartbeat. I had to sometimes hold the probes in such funny positions! It became quite tiring and uncomfortable sat in one position for that amount of time. They were certainly cheeky little twins already!

I was also struggling with my gestational diabetes. Again, due to Covid, it wasn't easy to get the food I needed on the ward. The main meal, lunch and dinner were fabulous, but the breakfasts were difficult, as all food was brought over from the main hospital. With COVID restrictions, nothing hot was being prepared on the ward, which meant the options included cereals, toast, yogurt and fruits.

As a coeliac requiring a no sugar, low carb diet, it was a challenge. The staff managed to find gluten free bread and cereal, but without protein, my levels were struggling. Plus, carrying twins, I was needing snacks in between meals, which really needed to be protein. I think some mistakes were made and my tummy was struggling, which wasn't helping, as I experienced tightening due to wind. Pete was great in getting lots of food in to me to help, but sadly, this was about to stop.

28 Weeks, 6 Days Pregnant

The first major 'Covid change' to our ward happened on Sunday, 29th March. The ward required a 'Covid-protected area' in case any mums arrived 'positive.' It meant they were shutting off half of the ward and there would be one antenatal ward (of four beds and a private room), next to the postnatal rooms. We would have to use the toilets in postnatal now (and the nearest ones were shut due to refurbishment. With Covid, that refurbishment had to be held off, too!) I had to leave my protected private room to go on a ward of four.

I was very nervous with everything happening around me, alongside the looming realisation that Pete might not be able to stay with me for much longer. It was an upheaval having to pack up all my things and move again when heavily pregnant. With permanent steroids for my asthma, and having previously suffered for three years with severe ME that had left me wheelchair bound, it was scary to think about Covid. Whilst I was now very much recovered, I still suffered badly if I caught any infection or viruses. I was also missing my Sebastian terribly! It was hideous. I think all of this led to my next 'false start' labour that night, when our second miracle happened.

Labour number 2

That night I was feeling unwell, but I just put it down to the worry and dietary issues I was having. My second CTG was OK (just long as usual). Pete then left for his accommodation. Shortly after, I started to feel tightenings, so they put me back on the CTG and it showed that I was having moderate contractions again.

After monitoring for a while, it was decided I needed to go straight back down to the labour ward in case I needed an emergency caesarean section. I phoned Pete, and he rushed back. We had a wonderful midwife, who took over and strapped me up to the CTG again. They put two cannulas in. By this point, I was pretty used to being prodded and poked. I am not squeamish. However, I do hate cannulas! (*I have very small veins with bony hands and arms, so they always struggle to get cannulas in: they tend to go on the side of my wrist or elbow. It hurts, and I'm like a big baby who just wants them out!*) However, I pulled up my big girls' pants and carried on.

I was injected with something called magnesium sulphate and given steroids to help mature the babies' lungs. Magnesium sulphate is given to mums under 30 weeks pregnant, as it reduces the risk of cerebral palsy and it protects gross motor functions in preterm babies. Magnesium sulphate is a funny thing: it makes you feel really, really hot all over (especially down below), which I found hilarious. The downside was that it caused a searing pain in my arm, but I think that could have been related to the cannula position. I had to keep it on until they were sure the labour had subsided again, which luckily it did, so by the morning I could relax again. The babies weren't coming yet!

It was during the night that our second miracle happened.

Our wonderful midwife listened intently to our story. It just so happened that she had a friend (who also used to be a midwife at Princess Anne), who wasn't able to travel back from New Zealand because of Covid restrictions. This friend, therefore, had an empty, furnished flat just down the road from the hospital. The midwife said she would immediately contact her friend in New Zealand to see how she'd feel about Pete moving in, and then once the babies were born and I was discharged, I would also join him (as it would be near the neonatal unit). Even better, Sebastian could then come and be with us, so we'd all be reunited!

The lady got back to us very quickly, and Pete was able to move in the next day! It was amazing. She only wanted bills covered: she would let us be rent free. We couldn't believe it! There was finally light at the end of the tunnel for when we would be reunited as a family again. This generous gesture helped me to keep going, even on the dark days to come. Even though I could be alone for another three weeks or so, I now wouldn't be without Sebby for another twelve. It really was a kindness that we would always be so thankful and grateful for.

The dark day

29 Weeks Pregnant

My labour had stopped and I would be going back to antenatal. That's when our poor midwife had to give us the news that Pete was no longer allowed on the ward.

Once we left the labour suite, we didn't know when we would be together again: both of us would have to go through the next part alone. As you can imagine, it was devastating. I was scared and sad. I wanted Pete; I wanted Sebby; I wanted my mum. It was cruel.

Sidebar: *Pete and I met late in life. I was thirty five and he was thirty seven. We'd met on a blind date set up by a mutual friend. It really was a meeting of two souls: I'd never believed in soulmates until I met Pete, but here it was: love at first sight. We were married within seven months of meeting on May 29th, 2015. We had a wonderful wedding day filled with all our nearest and dearest. Having been poorly for so long, and only starting to recover in the March of that year, I never dreamed I'd meet someone—let along be able to walk down an aisle. It's crazy how things can change so quickly in life. You just never know what's around the corner! We are a strong couple, who are lucky enough to love each other very much and be each other's best friend, as well as partner. Some of you may feel like throwing up... but without this kind of bond, it would have been even harder to get through what was coming next.*

The staff kept us in labour suite for as long as they could, so Pete and I could have some time together before we had to say goodbye. We just cuddled, then he helped me have a bath and clean up. Just the normal, everyday things were about to be taken from us that we all take for granted. Then the time came; they wheeled me up to antenatal and we said goodbye. I was a mess—I am as I write this. I cried and cried. I wanted Pete! How could those making these 'rules' think that this was good for the health of a heavily pregnant mum in a dangerous situation? I don't know. You could see the pain in the eyes of the hospital staff, too: it went against everything they stood for.

The strange thing was, once Pete had gone, a strength came over me. I had to carry on. I had to stay calm for my babies; I had no choice. As they wheeled me to my bed, there was another mum opposite, who had also just been told she had to stay in without her partner. We cried together, but we also chatted and found strength together with an instant bond of support. The midwives were amazing. They came and sat with me and talked. They were to become my support and 'my partner.' The other mums were to become my friends.

Reflecting back, I feel for Pete as he had no one. He was on his own in a flat, not being able to see people because of Covid, and he just had to wait. That must have been horrendous. I mean, I'm not saying I had it easy (!) but at least I wasn't alone, and in these kind of situations, strangers become friends.

On my own

I settled into a pattern of my very long CTGs, eating, speaking with Pete, Sebby or my parents, and chatting with the girls on the ward. It quickly became apparent that it was quite a quick turnover in antenatal. People would come into the ward in the early stages of labour, and then be moved down to the labour suite. Other people with fetal issues would come and, if they lived nearby, be allowed home or have short stays.

I was in it for the long-run, but it kept me strong by being able to share my story with these ladies. In turn, I would hear their stories and give them my support by telling them that if I can get through it, then they can too. I'm not saying I felt positive every day. I didn't. I missed my family terribly and I felt scared, but I had to carry on: I didn't have a choice.

The staff couldn't have been more amazing, particularly a couple of student midwives who were such a support to me. They weren't just there for our medical needs; they became our confidants, our daily contact and comfort when we needed it. They had to be everything. It must have been very hard for them, too.

Sidebar: *Everyone talks about the happy side of giving birth and babies, but infertility and complicated births aren't highlighted enough in my opinion. During my time in antenatal, I was surrounded by women who had been on all sorts of journeys to get their babies. Many of the women I spoke to thought it would be so difficult to either 'get pregnant' or 'stay pregnant' and struggle throughout. None of us thought we are going to be the ones with serious conditions, either.*

I mentioned earlier that I'd had problems conceiving Sebastian, so I had some idea of what it was like to want a baby badly. We tried for Sebby for what seemed like an eternity. We started trying for him as soon as we were married, and it took two years and five months before we met our beautiful son. When I was poorly, I had moments where I never believed I would meet someone, let alone have a baby. I'd always wanted children. Because of our age, we started trying quickly, otherwise we would have waited a little while. After a year and a half of trying, we both went to get our fertility checked and it seemed we were both OK. It's what they call 'unexplained infertility.' I had my tubes flushed to check for any blockages. This was a very upsetting experience for me. Although a quick process, it was very painful and it felt like another blow to my already low mood at the time. However, within three months, we were pregnant with Sebby. Whether it was a coincidence or there had been a blockage, we will never know. Apparently, it's well-known for 'the flush through' to work, which is why consultants wait three months afterwards until any further treatment. We were ecstatic: our baby was finally on his way and my dreams were being delivered. Literally!

I was so lucky. So many women (including friends of mine) have suffered horribly with infertility, and I don't think until you've been in that situation, you will ever understand the pain it brings. These women deserve our support, kindness and understanding. It seems so unfair to be unable to do what some people seem to do so naturally and quickly.

Being on a ward surrounded by amazing mummies, I'd never dreamed that I would be part of this gang. Yes, it was painful and difficult for us all, but we were also strong, brave women—some going through unimaginable pain—yet we laughed together. Everyone was supportive and kind. I think it would be hard for anyone to really understand this unless they have been through it, but I hope I paint a bit of a picture.

I was still struggling with my gestational diabetes and getting the right food. One of the student midwives was allowed to go to Marks and Spencer's and get various gluten/wheat and sugar free snacks to help my tummy. This was such a kind gesture, and a small way to show how the staff really would go above and beyond for us ladies if they could. Plus, the catering staff were brilliant with giving me extra yoghurts, fruit and anything they could! The meal menus were well thought through, so I was able to eat well for lunch and dinner. I have to say, though, I really could have done with a massive sponge pudding and a big bar of chocolate rather than an orange to comfort myself! It really was a small price to pay for keeping me and my babies well, however. I have an even greater respect for people with diabetes after living a few weeks in their shoes!

I want to add that, due to Covid measures, the student midwives were given the option to go home or to stay and be away from their families. So many of them chose to put aside their own comforts and stay helping—a very hard decision—especially when some of the students were as young as nineteen. A lot of student doctors and nurses also made that decision to help on the wards (rather than go home) especially at night, as staff levels were struggling with people off shielding, isolating, poorly, or called out to work in intensive care. We often had a young trainee doctor or nurse doing our stats and generally helping out. These are definitely some of the hidden heroes of the pandemic.

Mums of young children will understand how hard it is to get them to talk for any great length of time on video chat or phone. I devised a plan to draw a picture for Sebby every day, and then be able to chat with him about it when we spoke. This definitely helped. Possibly more for me, as it gave me something to focus on that I could do for him, even though I was so far away. I'm not a great artist, but I decided that I wanted to try and I actually really enjoyed it. It helped rest my mind and it was something to do other than TV or audiobooks. Sebby was still doing brilliantly with my parents. They settled into a routine that kept them all very busy. I will forever be so grateful to my mummy and daddy for having my precious boy for so long, and being his everything whilst I couldn't. Just to add, they are both in their early seventies, so this was even more of an amazing feat to suddenly have to parent a two-year-old full time. Just to know Sebby was happy and safe meant a lot to me, even though it was incredibly hard. We explained as much to him as we could, but we will never know what he really thought or how it affected him. To be suddenly taken from your parents, however loved you are, must still leave its mark.

Covid-19 was being utterly cruel to the whole hospital. When I told you they had to change the antenatal ward around in case of an influx of infected mummies, I didn't go into the details of how this affected us on antenatal. I explained that we had to use the toilets in the postnatal ward, which meant a walk along the corridor past all the new babies and parents. On top of this, our antenatal room was next door to the postnatal rooms. We weren't allowed to see our partners, but in the room next door, partners were allowed in once the baby was born. Mentally, this was hard to comprehend. Due to Covid, we had to be alone, but literally a few feet away, the partners were there. It didn't make sense. I'm just so glad for the mummies that (after labour) the partners were allowed in, because this wasn't the case in all hospitals at this time. This was long before regular testing was on offer.

The other hard bit was the joy, but also the sadness of hearing healthy baby cries. I felt elated for the new mummies but also incredibly sad, as we were desperately fighting for our own babies' lives. If it wasn't for Covid, this wouldn't be allowed to happen. It wasn't fair, but none of this was fair. It was just life, and life can be hard. The hospital had no choice.

It's going to snow

29 Weeks 3 Days Pregnant

The following Thursday, 2nd April, I went down to Fetal Medicine for MCAs to be checked and I had my full scan of the babies' sizes. The babies were growing well and the MCAs were still looking good. Leo, however, was starting to show signs that he may not want to stay put for much longer. I was now 29 weeks, plus 3 days, so we were doing well. I was infection-free, but I was definitely starting to feel very tired and not quite myself.

The staff explained it to me by saying 'it's going to snow.' They said that you look out of the window and it's currently sunny, but snow is due; the clouds are building. It could be an hour; it could be days, but the snow is going to break sooner rather than later. Leo wasn't showing any signs of distress, but it could change very quickly. We just had to keep monitoring. They decided to book me in for another scan on Monday and see how the weekend went.

I went back to the ward exhausted. I showered, washed my hair and changed my clothes. Every time I went out of the ward I was in danger of bringing Covid back in, so I had to be so careful: not only to protect myself, but everyone else, too. I rested, spoke to Pete and Sebby, cried, ate, and chatted with the ladies. I had another CTG that took hours again, and just tried to sleep.

29 Weeks 4 Days Pregnant

The following day I had to be taken over to the main hospital to have my MRI. This was the MRI that I was supposed to have at St. George's, to check for neurological damage that TAPS may have caused to the babies. However, because my waters had broken, I couldn't go up to London, so the fetal medicine department organised for me to have the MRI at Southampton.

I was quite nervous about it, and I wasn't feeling great in myself with everything that was happening: the gestational diabetes; my thyroid levels had changed; being coeliac, and being heavily pregnant. I was beginning to feel even more alone, even though I wasn't physically. I missed Pete terribly. My lovely student midwife came with me again. We had to get a taxi from one side of the road to the other and then walk to the MRI, which was on the ground floor of Southampton Hospital. Again, people couldn't have been kinder.

Going into the main hospital was slightly nerve-racking, as this was during the first peak of Covid and everyone was still so unsure of it. We all had masks on and, what was usually a bustling main hospital entrance, was pretty much deserted. It was very strange. It was the first real experience of 'Covid and the real world' outside of my hospital bubble in over a week. Things had changed dramatically. I'd obviously been reading the paper, but to see it first hand was very different.

For the MRI, I had to undress and put a gown on. I was taken into the room where the staff made me as comfortable as they could (on my side, using various props). I had to put on protective headphones and keep very still. The details feel slightly hazy now, but it was at least thirty minutes long and I had to go into the MRI scanner fully. It was loud and not the most comfortable thing for a pregnant lady, but I used a processing tool to imagine myself somewhere safe and happy. It helped a lot.

Once back in the ward, I showered and washed my hair again. I was feeling shattered and uncomfortable; the last few days had taken their toll emotionally. I missed Pete and his support terribly. It just wasn't the same seeing him or Sebby on video chat. I certainly had a few tearful moments. I cuddled down in bed and tried to rest until my CTG.

Labour

I didn't feel well all afternoon but put it down to having had an emotional, and physically challenging, couple of days. I'd been alone now for five days, and without Sebastian for a week and two days. It doesn't sound long, but when you are going through something so hard on your own, it feels like months. It's the 'not knowing how long it will last.'

I knew that the longer the babies stayed in, the better, but it was getting physically more difficult for my body each day. It was also quite terrifying to think what could or might happen. I still had no idea how the twins would be born. Would they be ok? Would there be repercussions from the TAPS? If they came soon, then would they be big enough and strong enough to survive? All these questions and more. I tried very hard just to think in hours and days, and not think too far ahead, otherwise it was just unmanageable.

That night I had my CTG. All seemed fine, but I just wasn't feeling well. Later on in the evening, I explained to the staff on duty that I felt tightening in my tummy, like mild contractions, and I just didn't feel right. I couldn't sleep. It hadn't been picked up on the CTG earlier so I just presumed it was coeliac symptoms. They strapped me up again to the CTG and this time there were small contractions starting. They weren't too concerned yet about the babies, but worryingly my heart rate had started to increase and it just wasn't coming down. I was feeling quite unwell. They quickly decided I needed to be monitored in the labour ward. It was around 3 am. Pete was called and told to meet me there. I remember that night there was a lovely student nurse on: he'd been the one to closely monitor me and saw things weren't right. He was only twenty one, but he packed up all my things and made sure I was ready to go. He was so kind: I obviously wasn't in a position to do anything myself.

29 Weeks 5 Days Pregnant

Once in the Labour suite, everything went very quickly. The CTG showed that Leo was also now in distress: his heart rate kept dropping and my heart rate was not coming down. I was 29 weeks, plus 5 days, and although ideally we needed to keep the babies in longer, it looked like my body—and now Leo's—had other ideas. I have to say, I did feel like this was it. I felt different. I knew that I couldn't keep going any longer, and the babies needed to be born. It was all taken out of our hands very quickly: Leo's distress was increasing. The babies had to be born—and quickly. The cannulas went in and the magnesium sulphate started. I was put on stronger antibiotics, injected with anti-sickness medication, and then quickly taken through to theatre.

Pete had arrived at the hospital around 4am, but as soon as he'd arrived, it felt like I was being wheeled away from him again to theatre. I remember I kept saying to the nurses: "Where is my husband? I want my husband!" and it felt like an *age* until he finally came in, wearing scrubs to hold my hand.

They'd already begun the procedure. I'd had a spinal anaesthetic again so was fully numb from the chest downwards. Once the contractions started, I had to hold very still so they could put the needle in my back (which is a feat when in pain). Previously in the labour suite, I'd said to Pete: "I'm not meant to be having contractions; it's meant to be planned and easy. I didn't sign up for this." It was the rant of a scared, pregnant woman, who very much remembered the twenty-eight-hour labour of Sebastian!

Again, the theatre was full with people. They had to have two sets of everything. Two midwives, two nurses, two surgeons, and two neonatal teams for when the babies were born. It was very busy, and everyone was focussed: you could tell this was a serious situation.

The anaesthetist was in charge of me, talking me through what was happening until Pete arrived to hold my hand. I was feeling very poorly indeed. The magnesium sulphate, mixed with the adrenalin of the situation and a possible infection, meant that I couldn't stop shaking (made even harder when paralysed). My teeth and jaw wouldn't stop moving: it was painful, and eventually I started to be sick as well. They put a screen up so I couldn't see what was happening, but they did shout out each time a baby was born.

At 5.36am, on Saturday 4th April 2020, Asher made his appearance, weighing two pounds and ten ounces. Leo followed, who had apparently tried to escape so was harder to reach, at 5.39am, weighing one pound and fifteen ounces. Both babies were intubated and taken straight to neonatal ICU. Intubation is where a tube is inserted into the babies' airways so they can be placed on a ventilator to aid breathing. At this point, my babies were unable to breath on their own. They had to work on Leo for a lot longer than Asher, as Leo wasn't alive when born, but they got my baby back. Both boys were alive and pink! A miracle. We'd survived TAPS as far as the blood was concerned, and now it was time for our neonatal journey to begin! We still had a long way to go, but both boys had arrived!

Babies are here

Then the next evil happened due to Covid. The boys—being so small, and Leo so unwell at birth—were taken away very quickly, and neither Pete nor I were able to see them. Due to Covid restrictions, there was a 'one parent rule' per child in the neonatal. Even though we had two babies, we still counted as one family. I would be the only person able to visit them.

This meant Pete would not get to meet his baby sons until these restrictions ended, and that might not be until the babies came home. This was a devastating blow to Pete. We'd prepared for the fact he wouldn't get to see them in neonatal, but we had been told (and hoped) that he would at least get a glimpse of them at the birth, just to be able to say hello to his baby boys. Unfortunately, due to circumstances out of everyone's control, this wasn't the case. Pete had to deal with the fact he wouldn't see them for a good while, and I had to deal with his pain, as well as the fact that I'd have to 'go it alone' on the next part of our journey again.

The upside was that Pete was allowed on the postnatal ward, so although he wasn't able to see the babies, he could be with me. This was amazing. Initially, I was wheeled back to labour suite for monitoring. We were told the babies would be settled in NICU and, when I was a little better, they would wheel me through on the bed to see them. I remember being in a bit of shock that they were born. I was excited that (so far) they were OK, but I was also in pain for Pete.

Physically, I was still completely numb from the waist down so was comfortable. Once all the drips had stopped, the sickness stopped and then I started to feel better. Another small and silly thing that brought me comfort was that I could finally have the hot chocolate I'd craved since my gestational diabetes diagnosis! Once the babies were born, I could go back to normal, as the illness usually subsides. That hot chocolate was the best I've ever had!

We phoned my parents and Sebby to tell them the news. It was my mum's birthday, so we had an extra special present for her. Two new grandsons! Both my parents were overjoyed. I think they were somewhat relieved that I didn't have to be alone anymore, and that my body could now heal, as well as the great joy of the boys being born and alive. *You never stop being a parent, however old your child is. I'm very close to my mummy and daddy and it must have been very hard for them not being able to get to me or see us. I think the focus of having Sebastian to look after helped them a great deal.*

At around 11am, I was wheeled into neonatal. Again, due to Covid, I'd never been in the unit before. Generally, parents are given a tour, but I had seen it on a video. I knew there were four rooms: Two NICU (Neonatal Intensive Care Units,) a HDU (High Dependency Unit) and a large SCBU (Special Care Baby Unit). *Babies go into whichever room is suitable for their level of care and then move up as their situation improves.* My two babies were in NICU 4, as they were extremely premature and were ventilated. At 29 weeks, plus 5 days, we had come a long way. A lot of singletons born at this age would be considered premature (rather than extreme) as they tend to be born in the three pound category, although every situation is obviously very different. However, with twins, they are a lot smaller. Even though they'd reached this great milestone, they were much smaller in size—more like the 25/26 'weekers,' so it made them extremely premature, especially Leo. Thank goodness they'd got this far: imagine how small they would have been even a week before.

Neonatal

1 Day Old – 29 Weeks, plus 5 Days

Getting used to going into neonatal was the next hurdle. I was wheeled into the boys' room, where they were inside two incubators diagonally to each other, with two other babies in between. As a parent, it's quite a frightening experience. There are a lot of machines, a lot of beeping, a lot of tubes and you are faced with very sick babies: it's hard. I had the joy of meeting my two little ones with the reality that they still weren't out of the woods yet. It was very daunting to think that I was going to deal with this new scary world of neonatal.

The staff couldn't have been kinder with their wonderful sense of humour and care. Due to Covid, everyone was masked up and wearing PPE (personal protective equipment) which consisted of aprons and gloves on top of their uniforms, so even though I couldn't see full faces, their eyes said it all.

Each baby had their own nurse. I saw Asher first, then Leo. They were both ventilated and had heart and breathing monitors. They were attached to all sorts of miracle machines to give them exactly what they needed.

The incubators are there to 'recreate' the womb. The babies are kept very warm and cocooned, being fed all the vitamins and nutrients they would be getting from the placenta. They have cannulas in for any antibiotics, and something called a 'long line' to help get things quickly into their systems. There is a lot more to it than this, but as a mum, this was plenty of knowledge.

Looking past all of this, there were two perfect tiny babies, with ten fingers and toes each. Everything was perfect—just so small. I was amazed. I didn't know what to expect. Pete and I had googled '28 weekers, 29 weekers' etc. just so it wasn't such a shock, but when faced with the reality, it's very different.

I only stayed with them for maybe half an hour before I was wheeled back up to the ward. After all, I'd just had major surgery and was exhausted and needed to rest. The babies were safe. At present, it didn't seem that there was anything wrong with either of them. The TAPS so far seemed to have resolved itself, blood wise. We wouldn't know about the hearing or neurological development for a while yet, but now the battle was that they were extremely small and premature: they needed to grow and develop their lungs. It was explained to me that neonatal was a bit like a rollercoaster, where you'd always be moving towards an end goal, with lots of ups and downs on the way. Apparently 'boys, and twins' generally have a longer stay than girls or singletons in neonatal. They weren't out of trouble yet. My brave baby warriors needed to keep fighting.

Back up on the postnatal ward, I was well looked after. I'd been put in a postnatal room reserved for mummies whose babies were in neonatal. They knew how unkind it would be to put us in with mummies and their new babies. I was able to rest, but once the spinal wore off, the pain was excruciating! As I've explained before, I struggle with allergies to a lot of medicines and I find it hard to keep strong painkillers down. I thought I could get by with just paracetamol, but that was the worst idea I've ever had!! The midwives want you to get up and start walking as quickly as you can, and you have to learn to not use your tummy muscles at all. I was shocked by the intense pain, so I was very quickly on anti-sickness tablets and morphine. I did a lot of sleeping for the next few days. The morphine knocked me out. I also did a lot of eating sponge puddings—yay to sugar!

When you have babies in neonatal, it's not as simple as just breast feeding. Most premature babies can't start to suckle until at least 34 weeks (sometimes a lot later) and they need to be tube fed. I really wanted to breast feed, as I had with Sebby. I knew it was something I could do for my babies. If possible, breast is so good for premature babies, but anyone who's been through this will know it is hard. I had to initially hand express the colostrum (which is the initial thick milk that comes through) and then after a day or so my milk came in. I think where I breastfed Sebby up until a few months before, it really helped it come in quicker. I got myself into a pattern of expressing seven to eight times a day, then my milk would then be taken down to neonatal and frozen to be used for the babies. A feeding newborn would probably eat more like ten to twelve times a day (at least), but where mine were premature, I didn't need this quantity yet. I just needed to get my boobs working and keep them that way until the babies could feed.

Plus, of course, I had two to feed. It takes a while to start making larger quantities anyway and everyone makes different amounts. I was getting maybe 50ml a go, while other mums might get 100ml, but we mustn't compare ourselves: we are all different. Some mums make more when they feed naturally and will never get that amount when expressing. It was hard being strapped up to boobie pumps constantly, but knowing why I was doing it kept me going.

For these first few days, I would visit the babies for maybe an hour. I'd be wheeled down to the door of neonatal and then have to walk, as Pete wasn't allowed in. The neonatal unit was very big, so the walking was no mean feat after a caesarean. Soon after, I had to walk the whole way, as during the night there was no Pete and the ward was very busy. I had to walk my expressed milk down to be refrigerated. Also, if there was no one available to get me the sterilised equipment, then I'd express down in NICU. I was on floor E. Neonatal was on floor D. It was a five to ten minute walk. Due to Covid, the usual kitchen and use of sterilising on ward wasn't allowed. Covid really had a lot to answer for. However, the fact I had to keep strong for my little babies helped, and I stuck with the strict pain relief and got on with it. The babies were dealing with a lot worse.

When a baby is born early the most important thing is for them to sleep. So apart from doing their bottoms, keeping them clean, and feeding them (which is called their 'cares') it is very much about leaving them be. Their incubators are covered in big thick quilts to keep it dark for them and they are turned to make sure their little bodies don't get sore. They need to keep warm, sleep and grow. Just like they would do in my tummy. The nurses have computers for each baby and lists of exact times of feeding, medicines, changing. They are very strict with this.

It was slightly harder being a mum of twins. Due to Covid and Pete not being allowed in, I had to split my time between two babies that were socially distanced. I had to wash and gel my hands every time I touched either baby. The first week I spent getting used to everything neonatal entailed. For me, my main hurdle was emotionally getting used to going into NICU. My hormones were all over the place and, as all mummies will know, the "baby blues" can rear its ugly head from around day three. Sure enough the tears came and added to what was already a very tearful time anyway.

I remember feeling that I didn't know how I would cope with going into the unit day in, day out. How was I going to deal with all the pain and suffering around me? It felt unfathomable at first. I had a conversation with my mum, crying that I didn't know how I was going to get through. It wasn't just my babies: I was surrounded by poorly babies with operations happening all around. One of the worst things that happened emotionally was on day three or four. I got talking to another mummy (socially distanced) who had her baby in between Asher and Leo. The nurses and doctors can't give information about the other babies, and we weren't allowed to go near them, but a mummy can talk to another mummy. She told me her story, and how a few weeks before, she had lost her other baby—twin to the one here. Here I was, with two alive twins and she was in the middle of us having lost one of her twins. I was inconsolable. I couldn't believe that we'd been put together. I just felt her pain, and how unfair and cruel it was for her. On top of this, my boys were still very little, and it made it very real that I could still lose one or both of them. It was nobody's fault: the NICU beds are precious, and if a baby needs it they have to fill it. Thankfully for us both, after a few more days they were able to move her and her baby to the other room, so she didn't have to come into contact with us. I could see that her tears and pain had increased so much since we'd come into the ward. I will always be so sorry for our part in this pain and, even though I never got to speak with her again, I hope her baby and family made it through. I think of them often. While on the phone to my mum, this all came out. I remember her saying to me: "You are brave; you are strong, and today the babies are alive and here. You are their mummy. Take each hour as it comes, each day, and you will get through. They need you." So that's what I did.

Back to the flat and Sebby

5 Days Old – 30 Weeks, plus 3 Days

I was discharged from hospital on day five, Wednesday 8th April, and went back to the flat, which was a five minute drive from the hospital. I had my pain killers, anti-sickness tablets and injections for my tummy (all mummies have these injections after a caesarean to help stop blood clotting). You have to inject yourself for ten days.

Pete had made the flat as homely as possible. He'd travelled back to the island and got everything we would need: we were so lucky to have somewhere to call ours. I still missed my home though, and Sebby. We'd decided that I'd have a few days to recuperate before Sebby joined us, as I wanted to be a little stronger and brighter for him. I was still in a great deal of pain and very emotional. He was set to come on the Monday and we both couldn't wait.

I was going into neonatal twice a day, and coming home for lunch. This meant an hour and a half in the morning, and then the same in the afternoon. The time increased as I felt better and I would go for a few hours either side so that I could come home for lunch with Sebby and Pete, and then have time with Sebby before dinner and putting him to bed. Providing the babies were OK, we kept to this routine. Occasionally I needed to go in for longer. I constantly felt very torn between all of my family, wanting to be in two places at once. I hated leaving the babies in hospital daily and I hated leaving Sebby, as we'd been apart for so long. The nurses were always so kind: they reiterated that the babies needed to sleep and not be touched, so it was OK to not be there 24/7. They would look after them for me. Sebby, who was two, needed me as well. It was still incredibly hard though: it seems so unnatural to leave your children behind every day.

The day Sebby arrived was amazing, emotional and sad all at the same time. My parents travelled across with him and, due to Covid, we weren't able to cuddle my parents or go too near.

Sidebar: *I am very close with my parents; they are my friends as well as the people that brought me up. My mum is my best friend. When I fell very ill, I'd moved back home, and so for three years they became my full time carers. I don't think any parent expects to have their child back at the age of thirty-two, completely dependent on them. It must have been incredibly hard for them. Being a parent myself, I now understand the emotional 'pull' of having a sick child. You would give anything to take away their pain to make them better. The worry is constant. I don't think this changes whatever the age of your child. My parents had this for parts of my entire life. It must have been so difficult for them and very hard to not continuously worry. As you can imagine, we were very close. They hadn't been able to be there for what was the hardest thing I'd ever been through in my life— and that sucked!*

On arrival, we'd planned that Sebby would run to us, and then Pete would get the bags. I initially thought I'd stay in the flat, as the thought of not being able to hug my mum and dad was unbearable, but when they got here I just ran out crying! I had to see them. Sebby ran into my arms crying "Mummy!" We were all crying! It was a moment of great joy to have my baby back, followed by the harsh reality of having to go through this horrendous situation without my parents, and still not be able to go to them. Covid sucked! They left straight away, and I think I spent most of the day cuddling Sebby. We decided I'd not go into the unit that afternoon and concentrate on Sebby. We'd been parted for over three weeks and we needed that time together.

We quickly settled into a routine of me being at the hospital and Pete being with Sebby. I can't imagine how it felt for Pete not being able to see his children. It must have been awful. He dealt with it by focusing on Sebby, but you could see the pain it caused. Sebby was a joy though: a gorgeous happy two-year-old, who loved being with us in the "holiday flat" as he named it. He was so well adjusted after what had happened to him and was still happening. It must have been very confusing. Due to Covid, we obviously weren't able to see anyone else and, due to the babies, we had to shield. Pete's Auntie lived nearby and she would bring us care packages to the doorstep or extra shopping. Plus, there were other kind friends from the mainland and island leaving us bits or sending things. We will always be so grateful to everyone for making this time a little easier.

Meanwhile, the babies were fighting and growing. In the first week, we had our first rollercoaster dip when Leo had to have a lumber puncture due to an infection. *This is when they insert a needle into the baby's spine to collect some spinal fluid. This can then be checked for the type of infection and to rule out meningitis.* The warrior that he is responded well to antibiotics, and luckily the infection wasn't serious.

Then, after just over a week in the NICU, my brave warriors were moved to HDU—the High Dependency Unit. The babies no longer needed the intense care they'd had before, which was amazing. They were being weighed every other day to keep track. Leo was on and off his light machine for the first three weeks, as his jaundice levels took a while to stabilise. Asher was doing well in general, but did need a blood transfusion at two weeks old. This is very normal for premature babies, but still worrying as parents. We had two very stressful days as they couldn't get a cannula in him, as his veins were so small. They tried six times before a very strong nurse put her foot down. Asher's heart was not coping with it, and she guarded Asher overnight to give him a chance to recover before the doctors tried again the next morning. I made her promise to keep guard before I could leave the hospital. I did a lot of praying that night because, if it wouldn't go in, then they would have to put the cannula in his scalp. We really didn't want him to have to go through that. It was torture not to be with him and I was so worried. I phoned more than once to check on him. Luckily, the cannula went in the next morning and the blood transfusion was a success.

During your neonatal journey, there's a lot for mummies of premature babies to learn and get used to. Of course, there's the washing, bed changes and changing tiny little nappies, surrounded by tubes and wires, which is hard in itself. You realise your babies are tougher than they look: you can touch them and turn them.

Due to Covid, I wasn't allowed to hold our babies though; I didn't get my first cuddle until they were four-and-a-half weeks old. This was very hard, but I could put my hands into the incubators and hold them in there. It was decided that the risk to little babies outweighed the good from kangaroo care. I'm not sure I agree with that, as it's well known that kangaroo care/skin-to-skin (*when the baby comes and cuddles against your chest and hears your heart beat*), is known to really help premature babies develop and thrive, especially with their breathing. The nurses weren't even allowed to comfort the babies when we weren't there. It was very unnatural for them, too, and you could see it went against their instincts of helping these babies and mummies thrive.

The ward was a very different place before Covid. Usually, it would have been filled with mummies, daddies and siblings. There was a parents' lounge for the families to eat and give each other support. All this stopped because of Covid. The parents lounge was closed; no one was allowed in. The only time you did see both parents was if the baby was about to have an operation, then the parents got twenty-four hours to be together with their baby/babies. Or, if the news was bad, then both parents were also allowed in. In some ways, Pete and I felt lucky he wasn't getting to see them, as it meant the babies were doing well. The staff tried to support us as much as they could, even remotely by phone or email. *You have to remember we were in there as the first wave of Covid hit, and everyone was very frightened and knew very little about it. Since then, things have changed with testing being readily available, so I'm sure it's a very different story now.*

The hospital didn't have a choice back then and the staff had to follow the national NHS guide lines. It could have been worse, too; some units were only allowing mums in for a maximum of two hours a day. At least I could be with the babies whenever I wanted. They also encouraged us to phone regularly, even during the night: there was never a wrong time. If you wanted to check up on your baby then you could and should. I remember phoning at 3am, just because I was worried and wanted to check in. The staff also sent us photos and videos when we weren't there. This was a real lifeline for the parent who wasn't able to go into the hospital.

Pete and I never did understand why the 'one parent per child rule' meant we both couldn't be there. The same rule was applied for all multiple births up and down the country- one parent per family. Potty really, as it was very hard having to do the cares and comfort of two babies, eight feet apart. I never sat down. It was like doing the beep test at school every day, running laps between the two babies. Joking aside though, it made it harder and more exhausting. My recovery was certainly slowed by this process, but again, I did what I had to do and got on with it. The nurses were amazing and helped in every way they could.

Another major hurdle was learning how to feed little babies via tube. They are fed hourly at first: they start with a solution made up of all they would get from the placenta, and then slowly breast milk is introduced. This is supplemented at first with fortifier, which is basically calories to help them grow. When it comes to feeding the babies, they first check the pH levels in the babies' tummies—to make sure the milk is being digested—and that their acid levels are ok. Then, using a syringe, you feed the milk into their tube and thus into their tummies. It has to be done very precisely and gently, stopping if, and when, it affects the babies' breathing. At first, the nurses do this for you. When you are ready you learn, then you can be the one to feed your baby. It's not something you ever think you are going to have to do. I remember thinking I'd never manage it, but I did, and after a few weeks I was happily tube feeding them.

I think the scariest (but apparently very normal for premature babies) was the desaturations, bradycardia and tachycardia. Or, as we in the prem game call them: desats, bradys and tachys. So, what are these? In layman's terms: desaturations are when the babies' oxygen levels drop too low. Bradycardia is when the heart rate drops. Tachycardia is when the heart goes too fast. These can happen very regularly during those first few weeks. Sometimes, it might happen a few times an hour or more. The tachys seems to occur if the baby is in pain, cross or needing something, but the desats and bradys just occur as premature babies forget to breathe.

You have to remember they are meant to still be in the tummy, with everything breathing for them, so sometimes they just forget they have to breathe for themselves! It can also happen a lot when they are being fed. Being new to this, it was frightening when it first happened. The monitors all start beeping and the nurses rush to rouse the baby. If it's not too bad, they just need a little prod or tickle to remind them to breathe. If the saturation isn't coming up quickly enough, then they need extra oxygen, and in bad cases they have to be intubated. Even though you are told this is very normal, it still doesn't prepare you for it. I don't think you ever quite get used to it happening; you just learn how to deal with it.

Asher and Leo were both exceptionally good at doing all of three of these—and often at the same time as each other! Mummy here was frantically running from baby to baby, and I often needed help as, however hard I tried, it was impossible to be in two places at once.

The nursing staff were amazing. Staffing changed regularly, but you did get to know some of them. The High Dependency Unit (HDU) room was also lovely. It only had six cots, so it was generally very relaxed and I got to know another lovely mummy, which helped for support. We still had a breast feeding room, which was open to express, and have a drink or snack, but I mainly stayed with the boys as my time was precious with them. I did talk to other mummies, too. They were all brave, strong women with different stories to tell and very supportive of each other.

I really feel the neonatal journey needs to be talked about so much more than it is. I think it's a slightly taboo subject, as the thought of poorly or dying babies isn't a comfortable subject for anyone, understandably. It's so much more than that: these little babies are brave warriors—and their mummies and families too. These families need to be supported and it needs to be known about. Plus, there's many happy stories and joy from neonatal—many more than the sad. The process is hard for everyone, but there are lots of happy, healthy babies heading home. Those that don't come home need to be remembered, and their parents supported, so that they can grieve openly and talk freely.

We were in Southampton neonatal for two days shy of four weeks. Right from the start, we'd been told that we would hopefully be able to return to the island Special Care Baby Unit (SCBU). The boys had to reach certain criteria to be able to travel, as it was a long journey via ambulance—a good couple of hours. They couldn't be air lifted as they were too small. One of the main criteria was the boys' breathing. There were various levels of breathing help. Both babies were only ventilated for a few days, then they went onto something called Hi flow, then Low flow, and then 'off' (with a little extra oxygen into their incubators if needed). Different babies need different amounts at different times. It's very normal for them to come off for a few days, but then need to be put on again. Leo struggled more than Asher. Leo was on 'hi flow' and then 'low flow' for longer. Asher would come off for a day or two, but then need to go back on. Generally, this would happen with increased bradys and desats. If the babies were having increased feeds and struggling to digest or getting constipated, this affected their breathing.

Their little bodies had so much to deal with. If they needed the extra help, then it was important they got it. We were told, right from the start, that babies can go home on oxygen (or with breathing help) so there really was no rush. We had to do what was right for them. However, to be moved back to the island, at least one baby would ideally be 'off' breathing support, and certainly neither on high flow. The island services could deal with low flow and, once the babies were there, the local hospital could do what was necessary to help. The boys just needed to be ok to travel. We also didn't want to get there and then have to send a baby back due to being released too soon. That would be awful. Although we talked about it, we had no idea when it would happen, initially. But then it did! And all very quickly!

Going Back to the Isle of Wight

I remember broaching the subject about the island SCBU on Monday, 27th April. Pete and I might have to start paying rent from May, so we needed an idea of how much longer we would be in the flat. The owner was amazing and would let us stay for as long as we needed, but if we weren't going to be in there, then they rightly wanted to rent it out. We loved our "holiday home," and were very much into a routine, but we all missed home. We just needed a bit of reassurance we would get back there at some point. Sebby was amazing, but you could tell he missed his bedroom; his home. He'd been away from home for nearly seven weeks now and, although he was now safely back with us, it must have been very confusing for him. His world was the flat, the garden or the car. Mummy was backwards and forwards like a yo-yo to these mystery, never-appearing brothers. It's surprising what a two-year-old can deal with. He was an incredible, brave and strong boy. He still is... and the best big brother!

At the time, no one mentioned us going home. It was to be discussed between the Southampton and Island doctors, then they'd inform us of the plan. However, the next day I was told that the island was happy to have us back. The Island hospital were also happy to take both babies, even if one still needed more breathing help. It would all happen in the next two days. I was shocked and excited all at once! I explained to them that we would need to get our whole flat packed up (with help from our parents) to get us back to the island. If it could wait until Thursday, then that would be easier for us, otherwise we wouldn't manage. They thought this was ok, and explained that it was a case of seeing how the babies were with less breathing support over the next few days. When things were sorted, it would happen quickly, so we couldn't be told days/times for sure.

Each baby had to be transported separately, then the transport team would have to come back and do the whole process again. It was at least a four-hour process for each baby. Due to Covid, the ferries were only running every two hours and, due to the size of the babies, they couldn't be flown, so it would just take longer. Hopefully, one baby would go first thing, then the next baby would go in the afternoon, but possibly even the next day. That made me very tearful: again, I would have to decide which child to stay with, and which would possibly have at least a day without me. Plus, I would possibly be separated from Sebby and Pete again. They may even have to keep one baby longer in Southampton if their breathing wasn't stable enough. Due to Covid, Pete wasn't allowed in either hospital, so it wasn't like he could be at one and me the other. I just had to look to the future and hope everything would run smoothly.

We decided that (with the help of Pete's mum) we would move out of the flat, and book for us all to travel back on the Thursday. We would worry about what we'd do if one couldn't come back, if and when it happened. It was easier to work with the idea that all would be ok. If the worse happened, options would be daily ferry travel or *Air BnB*. Neither were something I wanted to think about. Travelling during COVID wasn't ideal when you all needed to shield. It was an anxious couple of days. Asher was doing incredibly well with his breathing, but Leo was still struggling.

Once the amazing Southampton transport team knew Pete hadn't yet met the boys, they organised it so that (once in transit) they would pause by the hospital entrance, then Pete and Sebby could first see Asher. Pete would hopefully next see Leo outside of St Mary's. This was so kind of them and gave us an extra incentive and excitement for going home.

3 Weeks and 5 Days Old - 33 Weeks and 3 Days Old

The day arrived, and whilst Pete packed us up, Grandma arrived to play with Sebby and then help pack the cars. I went off to the hospital to be with the boys. It was a very emotional morning. They took Asher at 10.30am and, as they'd organised, Pete and Sebby were waiting by the doors. The babies were transported in an amazing incubator; we called it a spaceship to Sebby! They had a neonatal doctor and nurse with them at all times. Asher was strapped down and covered, but Pete and Sebby were able to open the little door and peer in and see his gorgeous little self. There were a lot of tears and a lot of smiles. It was an amazing moment.

I then went back in with Leo, knowing Asher was in very safe hands. We had decided that I would travel back with Pete and Sebby on a 2.30pm ferry, hoping that Leo would then be on the 4.30pm ferry. If this didn't happen, then we would make plans accordingly, but after seeing the doctor that morning, we were reassured that St Mary's was happy to take Leo, even though he was still struggling breathing wise. The Doctor really thought that Leo was ok to travel, so it was just down to whether the transport team could make all the ferry timings and logistics. Otherwise, Leo would have to travel in the morning.

Keeping everything crossed, I left Leo at 1.45pm to go to the ferry. I was beside myself, even though I knew we would be reunited soon. Leaving your baby is the most unnatural thing to do. If I could have torn myself in two, then I would have. I wanted to be with all of my children.

The ferry journey back to the island went well. Pete dropped me off at St Mary's hospital, and then he and Sebby went home. Pete would come back later. By this time, it was 4pm.

I remember walking into the ward being very emotional and seeing Asher in our private room. Everyone was just so kind. They explained how everything worked in SCBU: masks needed to be worn, but otherwise things were the same as Southampton. It was currently quiet, so we had full attention, but babies can come in anytime. Then they asked if I'd like a cuddle. I looked at them, confused: *was I allowed?* This is when they realised I hadn't yet held the babies.

My first cuddle was amazing! Asher was still so little (just over 3lbs) and they put him down my top for skin to skin. I held him for at least half an hour, until he was getting too tired, and needed to go back into his incubator. It was such a special moment.

Leo arrived at the hospital around 6pm. The transport team managed to get back to get him, then make the 4.30 ferry. Pete was waiting outside of the hospital for his first glimpse of Leo. I was inside cuddling Asher, so I didn't get to see, but I heard all about it. He was a very proud daddy! Once Leo arrived in his spaceship, the staff settled him in, as I had to leave the hospital soon after to get Sebby to bed. It would be the first time back in our home for just under 7 weeks, so I wanted to be there for bedtime. Again, I had to leave my babies in hospital, but I felt confident they were in a lovely room and going to be so well cared for. After their long journey, they both needed to rest. I was told to expect them to possibly go backwards a little for a few days, due to the travelling, but they'd pick up again.

That night was a bit strange back in our home. I settled Sebby to bed and soon after went to bed myself. I loved being home, but everything did feel a little off kilter: I just needed to get used to my new routine between St Mary's and home. I'm naturally quite shy and very much an introvert (although on the outside I'm very good at fooling everyone). However, I can get very anxious and nervous, especially with new things and people. I just needed to settle into things.

SCBU

Due to having a caesarean, I still couldn't drive. We decided I would go for longer days with the twins, from 11am-3/4pm, now we were home. It meant that Sebby wouldn't have an undisturbed day, as I'd be able to be with him for longer periods in the morning and for dinner. It would also give me longer with the babies. We knew that as it was getting closer to the twins coming home, which meant I would be "rooming in" for a while, so Sebby would have to get used to me gone again for longer.

"Rooming in" is when the parent (or parents) live with the baby, but in the safety of the hospital, to get both parents and baby/babies ready for going home. The parents basically take over all the care, including getting used to any medicine, feeding, or breathing help they may need at home. Help is nearby if it's needed.

Whilst the twins still needed to sleep and grow (and not yet breast feeding), Sebby needed to be a priority—especially for his mental health; we'd already been separated for weeks before, and I don't think he entirely trusted I'd be coming back. Understandably, he was only two! Getting the balance wasn't always easy and, as I've already said, I felt pulled in every which way! But you do what you have to do to try make all of your children happy. Sebby also had his daddy at home, which made such a difference. They were very happy together. Pete was furloughed due to COVID.

The next morning, I was very much looking forward to my first cuddle with Leo. He wasn't quite three pounds yet and I couldn't wait to give him some kangaroo care. I'd been informed both babies were extra sleepy and their bradys and desats had increased due to the travelling. They needed to rest, but I was able to do all their cares, sing to them, and still have my much awaited cuddle with Leo, which was just wonderful. Asher was too tired, so we didn't push him. I happily pottered around their room setting it up how I wanted it, and I settled into expressing there. The hospital fed me very well, which was lovely, especially for someone who was always hungry—after all, I was expressing for two! I spent time getting to know the staff. It was a much smaller team than Southampton, so in the subsequent weeks I got to know nearly everyone, which was great. It was a six/seven baby unit, so it was really small and (I think because of this) babies thrived. Mummies were allowed to be so hands-on during Covid, because it was so much safer than in a massive ward with much more chance of the virus spreading. We still had to be super careful though, and all the strict rules were in place. At last, things were about to change for Pete, and he was finally going to be able to meet his boys properly.

4 Weeks Old - 33 Weeks, plus 5 Days

About 8.30/9am every morning, the consultants and doctors would do the rounds to check the babies and decide on any treatment plans. On the Saturday morning, one of the consultants (who had met us for the first time) realised Pete had never seen the boys properly. She was absolutely gobsmacked and couldn't believe it! She said that it would be ok to get him in for a few minutes that afternoon to meet them, and the ward manager agreed. We didn't tell anyone: the ward had no other babies, so it would have to be a secret. That afternoon, Pete came on the ward and met both babies properly for the first time. He was able to put his hands in the incubators to touch them and speak to them. Holding them still wasn't an option, but this was so much more than we'd been allowed and we'd take anything. It was a beautiful moment seeing father meet his babies, and really be able to take in their size and development. He was able to see for himself where they were, and that they were well. More than four weeks Pete had waited. I can't imagine the emotional toll on him from that separation, but finally it was over, and he'd met his babies properly.

I think this separation was one of the cruellest bits about Covid for us. Pete will never get those weeks back. He never got to see how small the babies actually were, or experience what it was like in neonatal. Luckily, Pete's a very positive, strong person; I think few would have coped as well as him. You also have to remember this all happened right at the beginning of the pandemic. There was no vaccine and no regular testing. Very little was known about the virus: rightly, everyone was very scared and on high alert. The hospitals had to be above reproach; none of this was their fault, it was the virus. Once regular testing could be offered and then vaccines, I'm sure it was a very different experience for parents. Thank goodness. We were just unlucky, but we (and the staff) did the best we could in a difficult situation. Whether it would be done differently if it all happened again—who knows. I'd like to think lessons have been learnt and that maybe now they wouldn't keep premature babies from their parents unless absolutely necessary. Only time will tell. What I will say to parents though, is that you will get through—you have to. It's surprising how strong you can be if you need to.

Within a week, the hospital changed the Covid rules and Pete was allowed to visit daily (never at the same time as me, so we had to juggle). Generally, I'd go in the day and Pete at night, but at least he got to see them. I wasn't alone in my neonatal journey now. Pete got to experience everything having premature babies entailed: the good and the bad. Like I've said before, getting used to desats, bradys and tachys isn't easy, but he got there. He quickly became a pro at changing little bums, and he got to have his first cuddles.

We settled into our routine. I'd get there between 10am and 11am and stay until 3/4pm, then Pete would arrive around 7.30pm for a few hours. My days were busy doing the babies cares, tube-feeding them, expressing, cuddles, and dealing with any new treatment plans or medicines. I'd also see the doctors and nurses. Double cuddles was something I experienced that first week, to hold both babies on you is just so special. They were both put into my top, and they happily slept on me for a few minutes. To smell both their little heads and hold them tight, my little miracles, it was worth the wait.

Both babies were doing well, but Leo was struggling with his digestion and therefore breathing. As the babies grew, their feeds were increased. Each time, Leo would find this a little harder and his desats and bradys would get worse. He was struggling with constipation. We'd managed to get him off 'low flow' after a few days of being at St. Mary's, but it was decided fairly quickly to put him back on. The occasional help of oxygen was needed—just to help his little body cope with the changes—and be able to eat and grow. It made a big difference to him. He was also put on omeprazole, which is an anti-acid drug. The doctors thought that, due to his struggle with digesting his food, this might be causing the desats and bradys as well. It could be that he was suffering with reflux. All of this helped him lots and he settled again.

One of the scariest things both babies did was stopping breathing whilst having cuddles. When it happens the first time, you do freak out a bit, but again you learn how to rouse them. If not, you receive help very quickly, so it becomes part of the normal premature experience. Although I never really felt used to it—it frightened me every time! As the babies grew, this decreased. By the time we came home, it had stopped, so it doesn't go on forever.

Another hurdle was both babies developing inguinal hernias: Asher bi lateral (so both sides) and Leo just on the right. It threw me a bit, as I just felt it was one more thing to happen to my gorgeous boys. However, I was told it was very normal for premature babies to get them, especially due to constipation. Treatment was an operation back in Southampton, but due to Covid, they weren't doing them unless necessary. They needed us to keep close eyes on the babies: if the hernias became incarcerated (trapped) they would be rushed over; if not, they would wait for the boys to grow a little, and it would be done in a few months. They were very tiny, so to go under anaesthetic now was much more risky. If it could wait, then that would be better.

As parents (even knowing it was routine) it was still frightening. Seeing the bulges on the babies, and having to be told what could happen in an emergency, fuelled my fear. Where we'd been through so much already, I took it quite hard. I just wanted the worry and pain to be over! I hated the thought of my babies being in any discomfort or danger. I just wanted to make it go away and make them all better. Thankfully, inguinal hernias aren't actually painful for the babies if they are not trapped—it just looks worse—and every time they get upset, they increase in size. I held on to the fact that it wasn't hurting them; hopefully all would work out. Being premature, there was still a slim chance (until their official due date June 15th) that the hernias might self-correct, so we had that to hold onto as well.

From 34 weeks, you can begin to start to try breast feeding. At this point, our babies were 4 and a half weeks old; they were still both under four pounds, and their mouths were tiny, so they weren't quite ready yet. We'd had a go, without success, so decided to try again in few days. I think it was around 35 weeks when Leo latched on. One of the nurses suggested to try a nipple shield, as this might help him lock on, and sure enough it did. He sucked away. It's very tiring for them at first, so you give them maybe ten to fifteen minutes, then top up with tube feeding. Depending on how long they were on the breast, I could decrease the top up feed. Where the babies were weighed every two days, it helped to gauge if they were getting enough milk. Asher locked on soon after, and I tried to give them one or two breast feeds when I was there. It did exhaust them though, and sometimes they needed to be left to sleep, rather than try.

One thing I haven't mentioned is their tubes! Premature babies become exceptionally good at pulling out their feeding tubes: it becomes a challenge, a badge of honour! The amount of time the nurses or myself would come into the room and find Leo or Asher waving their tubes around in triumph, as if to say: "*Haha, look how clever I am*." They did it with their breathing tubes too. It's potty really, as they hate having them put back in. You'd think they'd learn, but no… I think they must all be in a little club with scores to see who can do it the most times!

At around 35 weeks, we were moved into a room with one, sometimes two, other babies. The ward had become busy and they needed the room for a new baby coming from Southampton. Again, it was a little nerve racking moving from our cosy room to being with another baby, especially with Covid. You weren't allowed to move between rooms so we'd been very much cocooned in our own safe space. We quickly adjusted though. I made a lovely friend who I was able to lunch with and generally share the mummy ups and downs. We are still friends now. That bond you get from sharing this kind of experience never goes away. Very few understand, so you can create a close friendship quickly.

At around 36 weeks, premature babies tend to have a sleepy week. No one knows why, it just tends to happen. True to form, both babies didn't want to disappoint and did exactly this: it just meant it was a struggle to progress with the breast feeding, but it meant lots of growing for them.

Preparing to go home

6 Weeks and 2 Days Old – 36 Weeks

Also around 36 weeks the ward staff start to put together a 'going home plan.' Once babies hit 37 weeks, they are considered full term. The staff try to send healthy babies home from then, sometimes a little before. Asher and Leo were both doing incredibly well. They were both off any breathing help, out of incubators, and into a twin cot.

Asher had come out of his incubator at 34 weeks, plus 4 days, and Leo 35 weeks, plus 1 day. They were initially placed onto heat mattresses and their temperatures checked regularly to adjust. They were clothed and had around four blankets and a hat. They needed to become used to being in normal temperatures, yet being so small, they could still get very cold easily. Both boys adjusted brilliantly. They were still suffering with some desats and bradys, but these were starting to stop by 36 weeks. This meant that they could soon come off of the heart monitors and be put on sleep apnoea monitors for forty eight hours to be sure they were breathing on their own. Apnoea monitors register if a baby stops breathing for more than ten or twenty seconds (depending on how it's set) and lets you know if there is a problem.

I was aware that it was coming up to the time of "rooming in," so we could really progress with the breast feeding, but it was still a shock on Wednesday 20th May, when I was asked to start rooming in—there and then!

Unfortunately, a consultant—without realising—sprung it on me without the nurses having had a chance to discuss with me what was going to happen yet. I remember feeling incredibly upset, as although I knew the step was coming, it meant maybe another week without seeing Sebby. I felt I needed to prepare him, and the thought they needed me to stay, there and then, just wasn't comprehensible. It brought up so many bad memories. Due to Covid, once in the hospital, I wouldn't be allowed home until we all came home. As ever, the kind nurses talked to me, and a plan was made for the following day—if I could manage it—and if the babies didn't take to fully breast feeding after a few days, then we could stop. Then I could go home for a few days and then try again. The consultant later apologised to me. She hadn't realised that it hadn't been discussed with me yet. She was very kind as well, and explained they just wanted to help get me and the babies home, but there was no rush.

After speaking with Pete, we decided I would start the next day. The staff had decided we would stay on the ward back in my original room for a few nights, so I had their help. If that worked, on the Saturday Pete and I would go to the family room for a few nights to 'room in' together. Sebby would go to my parents. He wasn't allowed on the ward with me, but as the family room was en-suite (and in a separate area) Pete could be there.

I went home that night and spent time with Sebby. It was now dawning on us that our babies could be coming home very soon, which was both a fantastic and nerve wracking feeling. The thought that I had to leave Sebby again was awful. Even though it was just for a few days, it brought back all that pain of not seeing him for over three weeks, and the unknown of when I would. I was also acutely aware that I didn't want him to feel in any way abandoned. I wanted him to know that mummy was coming home. Both Pete and I were very nervous of him staying at my parents, purely because last time he'd been there he'd not seen us again for a very long time; we hoped this wouldn't trigger anything in him. We reminded ourselves that this was a very different situation, and that we were home, and Sebby would know that this was short term. He'd have his daddy and for one or two nights, his grandparents whom he loved very much.

6 Weeks and 5 Days Old – 36 Weeks plus 3

I spent a large part of Thursday at home and went into the hospital for 4pm. Leo had proudly pulled out his feeding tube again, so it was decided to leave it out for now, and see how he got on with boob and bottle. We'd managed to introduce a bottle of expressed milk recently with Pete, and it seemed like they would take it. The plan was boobie, followed by top up of an amount, dependent on how long they'd fed. We'd go from there.

The first night was horrendous: they both took beautifully to breast feeding, but with having to feed and top up each baby every two/three hours, I just wasn't getting any sleep. Plus, the little rascals kept pooing or being sick, so lots of bottom and bed changes. I quickly decided the next day that—during the night—it would be best to give one bottle of expressed milk, so that I could at least get a few hours of sleep, otherwise it just wouldn't be manageable.

That day was the Friday. We did well all day. Whilst Pete wasn't there, a nurse would help me with the top ups. Due to Covid, I wasn't allowed to go to the milk kitchen. I needed them to get me milk and bottles. If they were free, they would help me top up the babies as well. So with cares, cuddles and feeding, we were very busy. That night was much better: I got a tiny bit more sleep and the staff, who were so aware of how tired I was getting, helped all they could.

The next day our final Covid-related drama happened. Pete rang me explaining that Sebby was really unwell with a very high temperature of forty degrees. Generally, two-year-olds get bugs and bits, but with Covid around, it sent everyone into a spiral. There was no way of testing then, so it had to be considered that it was. *What did this mean?* We knew instantly that Pete wouldn't now be allowed to 'room in' with me. We knew that they would have to isolate myself and the babies—but for how long? Would they even let us go home? How was I going to manage, isolated in a room off the ward, with two tiny twins, with no help and not able to leave the room to get anything? I had to rely on the nurses when they could get to me.

Plus, most importantly, my baby boy was really poorly and I wasn't there! I wasn't allowed to leave to see him and, if I did, then I couldn't get back to the babies! I have to say, I had a complete meltdown! There were big snotty tears, a lot of swearing and shouts of, "I want to go home." I also managed to tip an entire hot chocolate over myself, burning my legs and causing even more upset, as I didn't have enough clean clothes (Pete was meant to be bringing me more when he arrived). A real "doh!" moment. Luckily, the most wonderful nurse (and someone who I will forever be so grateful for) took over. She cleaned me up and got mine (and the babies') clothes washed. She stayed with me throughout the change of rooms, then refused to leave, even when her shift ended—just to make sure we were ok, and I got the help I needed. Without her, it would have been a very different experience. I think she realised how vulnerable I was from everything we'd been through, then to hit this hurdle (at the final post!) just brought me mentally crashing down. I wanted to go home. I wanted my family. I wanted my mum, and I didn't want to be in hospital any more. Three months was enough. Plus, I was very sleep deprived—all of which didn't bode well to how I was feeling.

Sidebar: I'd suffered very badly with postnatal depression with Sebby. I tried to hide it for a long time before I admitted how I was feeling. When I found out I was pregnant with twins, it quickly became apparent it wasn't going to be straight forward. It was decided I would stay on my antidepressants and increase them if needed. I think, if this decision hadn't been made, I would have coped a lot less with everything. I was glad for the added help of the tablets.

Postnatal depression is a debilitating illness that can leave the mummy feeling great shame and a feeling of failure as a parent. On what should be a joyous time of your life, you can be left feeling lost, shut off, incredibly sad and sometimes unable to bond with your baby, amongst many other symptoms. Of course, like anything else, there are different levels of it. Everyone can suffer to different degrees. Women need to be supported and heard. It's another subject that really needs to be talked about more. Multiple birth mummies can suffer particularly badly, even with a fairly conventional pregnancy. Twins rarely stay put full-term, so a stay in neonatal is generally a given for a lot of cases. This can cause great pain and suffering for the parent and indeed parents. The dads can suffer too!

I'd had double whammy of a difficult pregnancy and then a long neonatal stay. I think, without the knowledge of postnatal depression from my previous experience and the help of the tablets, I would have really struggled to get through. As I write this, I know I've still suffered. I've had flashbacks and memories which have caused PTSD to a degree, but I've worked and am working through it. I mentioned at the beginning of the book that sometimes you can't polish a turd, and this is so true. Some days are just shit and you've just got to go with it. You know what? That's ok. Own it, say it, and don't be ashamed. You are a wonderful, powerful woman, who's given birth to a tiny human/humans: you're allowed to feel bad. It's ok to not be ok!

Once I'd calmed down and been told that, although Pete couldn't come in, they would be allowing me to go home once the babies were ready, I again pulled up my hot-chocolate-covered big girls' pants and got on with it! I now knew there was light again and we would still go home. I just had to get through the next few days: the babies had to show they could feed, put weight on, and not have sleep apneas. Challenge accepted: game on!

I'm not going to lie, it was hard being in a room with two little babies and no one else (especially at night) but, during the day, I just focused on feeding, resting or sleeping (when they slept) and holding on to the thought that we would soon be home. The boys were weighed on the Saturday. Although no gain, they had sustained weight. Apparently, this is very normal as breastfeeding uses up so many more calories. Providing they gained a small amount by the coming Monday, the consultants were happy for us all to go home! Asher had pulled his tube out on the Friday, and both babies were feeding well. They hadn't (as yet) had any apneas, so it was looking good. Night times were harder, as both babies were getting very hungry and waking often. Plus, there were a lot of poo changes and baby sick. This meant having to change the cot completely. I would have to ring the buzzer, wait for someone to be free to come, and then they would get what we needed and help me change everything (or top up the babies). As you can imagine, sleep was a rarity, but it's surprising what you can do when you need to. Lying next to my two beautiful babies was reward enough.

7 Weeks and 2 Days Old- 37 Weeks

Monday dawned and it was weigh in. My boys had done it! They were four pounds and four pounds six ounces. We hadn't had any apneas: we were going home! I was elated and scared all at the same time. After our long journey, we were finally going to be together as a family of five. The boys had survived Spontaneous TAPS and being extremely premature. There were now going home without feeding tubes, not on oxygen, and at 37 weeks (7 weeks and 2 days old). They had excelled! They had overcome and over-exceeded everyone's expectations. The boys had survived and, not only that, they'd done it in style. I had survived a horrific diagnosis, operations, separations, neonatal—and we'd all done this through the start of a world pandemic. If we could get through this, then we can get through anything!

Pete came to pick us up at 4pm. He wasn't allowed in, but comically (being on the ground floor,) I was able to pass everything (minus the babies of course) out of the window. The babies' last test to pass was a twenty minute check, in their car seats, attached to a heart monitor. This was to check they could sustain breathing in that position: it's something all premature babies have to be checked for. They passed. We were then taken to the door by one of the wonderful nurses. We had our medicines, our instructions of what the babies needed, and we were quietly wished goodbye. Another thing Covid robbed us of was being able to say goodbye to everyone on the ward alongside the excitement of the babies going home. Two other nurses popped their heads out to say goodbye, but it was a very different experience than it should have been. However, maybe it was rather apt: the babies had caused such a stir from the moment I got pregnant, to go home quietly without fuss was perhaps a good omen for the future!

On Monday, 25th May 2020, we got into the car and took our babies home. The moment that we'd only dreamt about was happening, and now life could really begin. We had three under three. A two-year-old and newborn twins. Life was certainly going to be interesting.

Moving forward

Of course, this isn't the end. I'm writing this three days before the boys' 1st birthday, and we've been through such a lot in the last year. We've overcome more hurdles; we've had little sleep; we've survived without getting COVID, and we've been learning everyday about our new twin journey, but that's a story for another day.

There were many reasons I wanted to write this, but the biggest one initially was to be that story of hope for other parents. When we were diagnosed with Spontaneous TAPS, it was a lonely journey. There was such little information out there: there tended to be research-based papers written for medical professionals, with frightening facts or a few scary stories of very sad cases. At the time, there was nothing I could grab hold of to keep positive or show there were success stories. I felt that—if we got through and were that success story— then I wanted to make sure we could share it, so no one ever had to go through that again. I wanted there to be information for parents that was clear and understandable. Most importantly, I wanted us to be a beacon of hope: the success story. If our babies survived, then yours could too: there is light at the end of the tunnel, and having this horrific diagnosis doesn't mean the end. Hope is so important for a parent: it's the one thing we can hold onto when all else is falling apart. Sadly, it can't always protect us from the pain. We were incredibly lucky: we were placed in knowledgeable hands that knew the syndrome, with professionals who were able to quickly act, and do everything they could to save our babies.

The awful truth is that a lot of babies still don't survive. Regardless of medical intervention, some babies are just not made for this world. However, there are many babies who could have been saved, if TAPS was known by every medical professional around the world dealing with monochorionic twins or multiple births, where babies are sharing placentas. A simple test of checking the MCA Doppler levels regularly in all of these babies, would help to save a lot of lives. It would also help to better understand how the condition develops over time, and when intervention is needed. Secondly, I urge all you parents in this situation to ask questions: don't be afraid to say the name TAPS. Knowledge is power; let's educate people to prevent unnecessary losses. I'm under no illusion that if my boys hadn't had a size difference and so were checked for TTTS and then monitored, the MCA levels wouldn't have been checked. I would very probably have lost both babies. This shouldn't and mustn't happen.

Thirdly, it's going to be about enabling and helping research for the future. Professor Asma Khalil, who saved our babies' lives, works hard at St. George's Hospital in London. She not only saves babies, but herself and her team of multiple birth clinicians run the first ever *Twins Trust Centre for Research and Clinical Excellence*, based at St George's, and enabled by the amazing *Twins Trust charity*. They are the people that will do the research to save and promote health in all multiple pregnancies. Without research, there's no way of knowing the future outcomes of syndromes and particularly TAPS. Being such a newly recognised disease, there's still no exact evidence of future outcomes for these babies. All that's known so far is that neurological damage and hearing impairment can affect some babies long term, and into childhood, but again—if the research is done and babies and children are regularly checked—the right treatment can be given. Then an idea of outcomes can be more readily available. There are obviously ways to help donate and fundraise, but maybe even more importantly: share your stories, talk about TAPS, push for help if you need it. Don't be afraid to speak out. Let's get this message out there and save lives: that in itself costs nothing and is invaluable beyond words.

I also wanted to highlight the multiple pregnancy journey and neonatal. A large' proportion of multiple births will need some form of neonatal care. I wanted to share my experience to help take away some of the frightening aspects of having a baby born early, and to really share what happens, so that it can help prepare anyone finding themselves in this situation. Neonatal is also not talked about enough. People shy away. As I said previously, I think this is due to the thought of poorly or dying babies being incredibly hard to talk about (understandably so). However, we do need to talk about it. We need to support the parents who have the horrendous losses, and we need to show that also great joy comes out of neonatal. With medical advances these days, there are far more celebrations than losses. Yes, it's hard and it's a rollercoaster, but these little babies are strong, brave warriors who can cope with so much.

They are fighters, as are all the parents out there who have gone through any of this. We keep going because we have to, faced with your biggest fear of the possible loss of a child or children. You have to fight; you have to have hope, and you have to believe you will come through.

At the back of this book, I have included a chapter on medical information of everything I've talked about, written clearly for parents to be able to understand if they have to go through any of the above or similar. Plus, there are some well documented websites for any extra advice.

Obviously, some of what my family and I went through, due to COVID, will hopefully never happen again to any of you reading this. That part of the story really is a "you wouldn't believe it!" Experiencing this through a world pandemic obviously made our story even harder, and perhaps that little more interesting to read. The pandemic situation has come so far in a year, with advances on knowledge and vaccines, so I really hope the future is looking brighter for everyone.

Lastly, I'd like to say another huge thank you to all the amazing people that work within fetal medicine and neonatal. You are all unsung heroes, who deserve so much more credit than I can possibly ever say! You are the cleverest, kindest, and funniest people I've ever met, with compassion and empathy coming out of every pore! You dedicate your life to saving and caring for babies, and their families. Thank you—from the bottom of my heart. I salute you! Thank you for reading.

TAPS

What is TAPS?

TAPS stands for 'Twin Anaemia-Polycythaemia Sequence'. This is a condition found only in monochorionic twin pregnancies. Anaemia means not having enough red blood cells (which contain haemoglobin, the red substance that carries oxygen) in the blood. Polycythaemia is the opposite—when there are too many red blood cells in the circulation. Small blood vessels can form in the placenta between the babies, connecting their blood supplies, allowing a slow passage of blood from one baby to the other. These are smaller than the connecting blood vessels seen in TTTS. This can cause the baby donating the blood (donor) to become anaemic (low blood levels,) and the baby receiving the blood (recipient) to become polycythaemic (high blood levels), which can lead to overload and strain on its heart.

TAPS can be more difficult to diagnose than TTTS, as there is no difference in the fluid volume around the babies. It can develop on its own, or after laser therapy for TTTS.

Who does TAPS affect?

TAPS is a rare condition that can affect monochorionic twins or more (with twins that share a placenta). It can occur spontaneously or following incomplete laser treatment for Twin to Twin Transfusion syndrome (see above). Small blood vessels in the placenta connecting the circulations of the two babies may allow blood to leak through from one baby (the donor) to the other (the recipient).

What are the warning signs?

The mother rarely has symptoms from TAPS—it is something that is detected on ultrasound scan of the babies. The Doppler scan measures how fast blood is flowing through the babies' blood vessels, in particular the Middle Cerebral Artery, one of the blood vessels in the baby's brain. If a baby is anaemic, the blood is thinner and flows faster. If a baby is polycythaemic, the blood is thicker and flows more slowly. If the Doppler scan finds fast blood flow in one twin and slow blood flow in the other, then TAPS is diagnosed.

What are the complications?

Because it is the red blood cells that carry oxygen around the body, the anaemic twin has to try harder to pump enough blood and oxygen around the body. If the anaemia is severe, this may lead to heart failure. Because the recipient twin's blood is thick, this can lead to blood clots (thrombosis) in the circulation; it can also lead to heart failure because the blood is harder to pump around the body.

TAPS is usually graded into 5 different stages; Stage 1 is the mildest form while Stage 5 is the most severe.

What care should I expect during my pregnancy?

TAPS is a rare condition, so you should be cared for in a Fetal Medicine Unit with expertise in managing the complications of twin and more pregnancies. Your twins will have regular scans, at least every 1 week. The Doppler blood flow in the twins will be measured. In addition, the growth and amount of water (amniotic fluid) around the babies will be measured to distinguish TAPS from TTTS or other complications.

What are the treatment options?

If you develop TAPS, your twins or more will be monitored regularly by ultrasound scan. If the health of either baby is affected by the TAPS, it may be necessary to deliver the babies early. If it's too early to deliver the babies, however, other treatments may be necessary; these include laser ablation, intra-uterine transfusion and exchange transfusion.

Laser ablation therapy

Laser ablation therapy involves finding the small blood vessels connecting the twins and closing them to prevent the flow of blood from one baby to the other. The surgery is conducted under local anaesthetic or an epidural/spinal, so you should be awake and, if you wish, able to watch the procedure and your babies on an ultrasound or television screen.

The procedure begins by inserting a needle and thin hollow tube into the fluid sac of one baby. The needle is removed before all telescope (fetoscope) with a thin laser fibre is inserted through the tube. The fetoscope finds all the blood vessels in the placenta that link the blood flow between the two babies. The laser is then used to seal these blood vessels. Each baby stays connected through its own umbilical cord to its main source of blood and nutrition; but the blood can no longer flow from one baby to the other through the placenta.

Intra-uterine transfusion

Intra-uterine transfusion (IUT) involves giving a blood transfusion to the anaemic baby while still inside the womb. You will usually be given a small injection of local anaesthetic in your abdominal wall to numb the area. Then a fine needle is inserted into the womb. The position of the needle is followed by watching it on the ultrasound scan. The needle is inserted into the anaemic baby's umbilical cord, and the baby given a blood transfusion through the needle.

Intra-uterine exchange transfusion

The polycythaemic baby's blood is too thick. If necessary, this can be treated by exchange transfusion. In this procedure, a needle is inserted into the polycythaemic baby's umbilical cord, as described above. Some blood is then taken from this baby. This blood is then replaced by a similar amount of saline (salty water) effectively diluting the baby's blood.

What might happen to my babies?
It may be necessary to deliver the babies early because of TAPS. If this happens, the babies may need to spend some time in the neonatal unit because they are premature. If it's too early to deliver the babies, another

treatment, such as Laser surgery, intra-uterine blood transfusion +/- exchange transfusion (see above).

How and when will my babies be born?
If the TAPS is mild, your babies may be born at the usual time, i.e. 36 weeks for twins. In this situation, vaginal birth may be possible, depending on other factors, such as the position of the babies. But if TAPS is affecting the babies' health, it may be necessary for the babies to be born early; in this situation, Caesarean section is more likely.

What can I do?
There is nothing active that you can do to prevent or treat TAPS. The most important thing is to make sure you attend your regular scans with the specialists who can detect TAPS if it occurs, and advise you on the best treatment.

TAPS information written by Professor Asma Khalil for Twins Trust.

For more help, guidance and information about TAPS visit www.tapssupport.com
Email- hello@tapssupport.com
and
www.twinstrust.org

Different Types of Twins

Fraternal twins two eggs; separate babies

Dichorionic / Diamniotic Twins (DCDA) two placentas, two sacs

Identical twins one fertilised egg splits and develops two babies with exactly the same genetic information.

Monochorionic / Diamniotic Twins (MCDA) share a placenta but have two sacs

Monochorionic Monoamniotic (MCMA) share a placenta and one sac

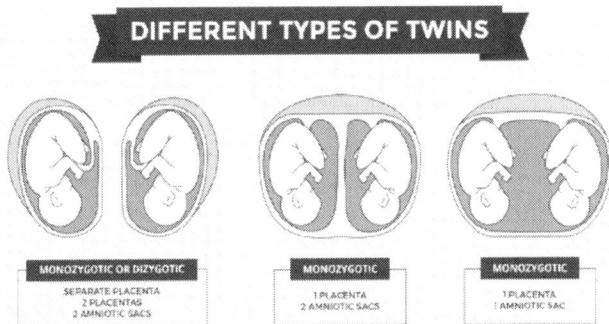

(Source Twins Trust)

Facts and Terms

All facts and terms are sourced through Twins Trust and researched by myself online. All checked and overseen by Professor Asma Khalil.

Anaemia Anaemia occurs when your blood doesn't have enough healthy red blood cells to carry oxygen to your tissues. Babies can become anaemic in the womb due to TAPS, TTTS, or other conditions and infections.
(Source Twins Trust)

Apnoea monitors monitors the babies breathing and heart. Sends an alert if baby stops breathing.

Breast feeding /Expressing / Bottle feeding this is a massive subject. All the information you will need is found at www.twinstrust.org. Here you will find detailed information and support to help you make an informed decision that's right for you.

Bradycardia when the heart rate drops too much.

Blood Transfusions in premature babies putting red blood cells back into baby to treat anaemia.

Caesarean baby/babies are delivered through a cut made in your tummy and womb. They are often performed if a natural birth would put the mummy or baby/babies in distress.

Coeliac a condition where your immune system attacks your gut when you eat gluten.

CTG (Cardiotocography) measures baby's heart rate and monitors for contractions.

Corrected age also known as adjusted age. It's the baby's actual age, minus the number of weeks or months they were born premature. For example, a one-year-old who was born two months early (before its due date) would have a corrected age of ten months old. Corrected age is used for the first 2-2 1/2 years of life. However, every child is different and the more premature the baby the longer it can take. Try not to compare your baby with others.

Desaturation when oxygen levels in the blood drop

Episiotomy An episiotomy is usually a simple procedure that involves a cut to the vagina and perineum (outside the vagina) to make more room for the baby to be born. A local anaesthetic is used to numb the area so you do not feel any pain. If you already have an epidural, it can be topped up before the cut is made. The cut is stitched together using dissolvable stitches after the birth.

Fetal Medicine Fetal medicine is the branch of medicine that provides care for the unborn baby/babies and mum. This includes looking after the growing babies growth and overall well-being, diagnosing and treating any fetal disorders. Looking after and supporting the parents.

Flush Through a doctor uses a liquid fluid, under pressure, to pass through the Fallopian tubes to insure that they are open and clear.

Gestational diabetes This is high blood sugar during pregnancy which is caused by your body not making/using enough insulin. Symptoms include feeling very hungry or thirsty, needing to pass urine frequently, tiredness and blurred vision. These symptoms are not always noticeable, hence the need for regular urine testing at antenatal appointments. Gestational diabetes shouldn't be a problem once it has been detected. Treatment involves dietary changes, close monitoring and sometimes medication in tablet form or insulin. It usually disappears immediately the baby(s) is born. The hospital will arrange a glucose test around 6 weeks after birth, to be certain that it has resolved. (Source Twins Trust)

Group Strep B
Group B strep is a type of bacteria called streptococcal bacteria. It's very common in women affecting 2-4 in 10. Group B strep is normally harmless and most people will not realise they have it. However it can spread to the baby during Labour and vaginal births and it can make young babies very poorly. If you are found to have it, they will give you antibiotics during birth and watch the baby closely afterwards. This is just to make sure there is no infection and treat if necessary.

GTN Patch / Glyceryl trinitrate used to help stop contractions and keep that baby/babies in! Also used to treat angina.

HDU (High Dependency Unit) babies still need advanced care but less sick than in NICU.

Heart Monitor keeps track of a baby's heart rate, breathing and oxygen levels.

Hi flow High flow oxygen therapy—breathing support for your baby. Oxygen, often in conjunction with compressed air and humidification, is used at a higher flow rate than normal breathing support to help your baby breathe happily.

Hypothyroidism your thyroid gland in your neck doesn't produce enough thyroid hormones. This can leave you with symptoms including fatigue, weight gain, sensitivity to cold amongst others. It's usually a lifelong condition, treated with thyroxine to replace the thyroid hormone you don't produce. If an under active thyroid is not treated properly during pregnancy, there is a risk of problems occurring. These include: birth defects, problems with the baby's physical and mental development, premature birth or a low birthweight, stillbirth or miscarriage.

However, these problems rarely occur nowadays as they can usually be avoided with treatment under the guidance of a specialist in hormone disorders (an endocrinologist). They will do regular checks of your thyroid levels during the pregnancy and adjust your dose of thyroxine accordingly. Then there is no concern for the baby. Don't be afraid to ask to get your levels checked regularly if you feel this isn't happening.

Incubator keeping your baby cosy and warm like they would be in the tummy. Simulating the womb.

Inguinal hernia is a small hole that has developed in the muscle in the baby's groin. This leads to some of the intestine poking out through this hole but still covered by the babies skin. They are quite common in premature babies. They usually require an operation.

Intubation a tube is inserted into the baby's airways to then be placed on a ventilator to aid breathing when baby can't breathe on their own.

Jaundice yellow baby—very common in new-borns. Can clear up on its own within two weeks but more severe cases need special light treatment, and occasionally an 'exchange transfusion,' where some of the babies blood is exchanged for new blood which doesn't contain so much bilirubin (the harmful yellow stuff)

Kangaroo Care "Skin to Skin " generally just wearing a nappy, baby is placed against mummy or daddy's bare chest. It has many benefits for premature babies including helping lactation and soothing both baby and parent and helping with breathing. More information can be found at www.twintrust.org

Low-flow Oxygen Therapy given through a nasal cannula. Supplemental oxygen to help breathing. Can be adjusted and turned down until baby is breathing air and needs no extra help.

Longline a fine plastic tube inserted into baby's small veins in their arms or legs to help reach a larger blood vessel usually near the heart. It prevents lots of cannulas and needles needing to be used on baby, which may cause stress. Helps feed them nutrients and medicines they need quickly and without stress to the baby.

Lumbar puncture A lumbar puncture (spinal tap) is performed in your lower back, where a needle is inserted between two lumbar bones (vertebrae) to remove a sample of cerebrospinal fluid. This is the fluid that surrounds your brain and spinal cord to protect them from injury. This test can be done for many reasons but typically to help rule out infection (meningitis)

Morning sickness a common symptom of pregnancy and includes nausea and sometimes vomiting. It can happen at any time of the day and be there all the time. It usually happens within the first four months of pregnancy but can go on throughout. People suffer in different degrees from mild to very serious called Hyperemesis Gravidarum.

MCA (middle cerebral artery) one of the main arteries that supply blood to the cerebrum (largest part of the brain)

Magnesium sulphate used in mothers delivering babies under thirty weeks to help project the baby's brain development or against brain damage caused by the babies prematurity.

NICU (Neonatal Intensive Care Unit) for babies that need the most amount of care.

Reflux when acid from your tummy comes back up into your oesophagus and throat.

Rooming in living in the hospital with your baby to get used to how it will be at home but with the support of the staff around you. Parents start to take back full control and care of their baby.

SCBU (special care baby unit) babies still need care, but are less sick or less premature than in other levels of care.

Selective fetal growth restriction Most twin, triplet or more babies will be slightly different in size, but sometimes one baby is significantly smaller than the other/s. This is called 'selective' growth restriction (sFGR)—when one baby is not growing at a normal rate. It can happen in multiples who have their own placentas (like dichorionic twins) and also in multiples that share a placenta (monochorionic) but the causes and treatment are different in each case. Selective fetal growth restriction occurs in 10-20 percent of monochorionic pregnancies when twins share unequal portions of the placenta. (Source Twins Trust)

Sonographer a person who specialises in using the ultrasound imaging device to see your baby in the tummy and check they are growing well.

Spinal anaesthetic an anaesthetist injects medication into your spinal fluid to numb you from the breast downwards. Often used for caesarean sections; also for laser treatment for twins.

Steroids used to help a premature baby's lungs develop—given to the mum (as two injections, usually 24 hours apart) when it looks as if her baby/babies might be born early.

Tachycardia when the heart rate goes too quickly.

Tube feeding babies that are premature or poorly are not able to feed with the breast or bottle. So a tube is inserted into their tummy and their food is injected straight into it.

Twin-to-twin transfusion syndrome (TTTS) is a rare pregnancy condition affecting identical twins or other multiples. TTTS occurs in pregnancies where twins share one placenta (monochorionic) and a network of blood vessels that supply oxygen and nutrients essential for development in the womb. (Source Twins Trust)

Ventilation baby is put on full breathing support with a ventilator breathing for them.

Printed in Great Britain
by Amazon